W9-AOI-974

The Health and Happiness of Your Old Dog

The Span of Life

The old dog barks backward without getting up,
I can remember when he was a pup.

—Robert Frost

The Health and Happiness of Your Old Dog

by George D. Whitney, D.V.M.

WILLIAM MORROW AND COMPANY, INC.
NEW YORK 1975

Inquiries should be addressed to William Morrow and Company, Inc., 105 Madison Ave., New York, N.Y. 10016.

Printed in the United States of America.

1 2 3 4 5 79 78 77 76 75

Library of Congress Cataloging in Publication Data

Whitney, George D (date)
The health and happiness of your old dog.

Bibliography: p.
Includes index.
1. Dogs—Diseases. I. Title.
SF991.W588 636.089'89'7 75-9826
ISBN 0-688-02949-3

Book design: H. Roberts

For Leon F. Whitney, D.V.M.

who was mentor, model and friend to a host of people, including his son.

Contents

The Health and Happiness of Your Old Dog

I
What's Your Problem?

Years ago, when I was new in practice and better prepared, I suppose, to be amused than instructed, a belligerent little man brought an amiable old dog to the office. He boosted the old fellow onto the table, fenced me back with his arm so that I could appreciate the stance, and shouted at me, "See! He's a stout old dog. And he'll live a long time yet." Then, turning to me with a gesture of helplessness, he added very quietly, as though he didn't want the dog to hear, "The only thing is, Doc—I'm afraid he's going to get old."

I don't think that the little man intended to utter a capital T Truth. But he did. That was a long time ago, but since then I don't remember having heard a more succinct statement of the hope-and-fear predicament of the owners of old dogs.

And it is a predicament, this Live-Long-But— dilemma. Everybody wants to keep his old dog as long as he can—and as well and comfortable as he can, as happy and pain-free as he can. And everybody—almost everybody—has a gnawing fear that he may not be able to accomplish all of that. He worries that he is not doing as much as he could or should to prevent or postpone the onset of the ills of age. He is afraid that as the dog grows older he will inevitably develop a series of increasingly painful and incapacitating ailments. And most of all, he fears that eventually both he and the dog will be overwhelmed by some final disaster that neither of them will be able to cope with.

For many owners this fear of the unknown future—and what other kind of future is there?—becomes a real problem. It is common. It is often painfully persistent. It is sometimes distressingly acute.

And it is a struggle with a paper tiger.

Old age in dogs, as in people, is something nearly undefinable. Your favorite dictionary will be of very little help to you. It explains incontrovertibly that old age is a time of life that follows another time of life described in equally vague terms. And wisely it lets it go at that. But whatever it may be, old age is not a disease. It is not a creeping calamity. And it is not an endless series of infirmities and disabilities.

Dogs are not devastated by age. Nor are their owners. The plain, observable fact is that dogs age remarkably well. The changes that they experience are those that are common to other animals—such as man. They slow down. There is a gradual reduction in activity, a decrease in energy and powers, a slow decline in the functions of some of the organs and processes of the body.

As they grow older, dogs do need—and should receive—an extra measure of care and attention. And always they should be protected against the hazards to which they are increasingly exposed as their responses become less quick and certain. But their aches and pains are no more severe than those of their owners—and often they can be more easily alleviated. The discomforts and disabilities that they may have are by no means unmanageable. They can always be treated and usually they can be cured or controlled. Old dogs don't totter off into senility and they don't become a burden to themselves or to their owners.

And whatever may happen to them, the time will never come—never—when a thoughtful owner will find himself unable to cope with the situation decently and humanely.

Owners often have to be reminded that this is actually a golden age for the family dog—far and away the best that he has ever known. And especially for the old dog. There was a time, more recently than you think, when by present standards all dogs were miserably mistreated. And Hector, far from being *good* old Hector, was no more than an inconvenient nuisance, scandalously and shamelessly abused. Whatever ills and infirmities he developed were assumed to be the natural and incurable afflictions of old age. He survived while he could and commonly died of untreated disease or was dispatched when he became so feeble that he got in the way.

Old dogs live well today. They are cherished and preserved and protected. They are comfortably housed and generously (too generously) fed. They are healthier and stronger and they live longer and more happily than they ever have in the past. Far from being outcasts, they have become the most privileged characters in every household. That's not quite heaven, perhaps. But it is close. Mark Twain said, "Heaven goes by favor; if it went by merit, you would stay out and your dog would go in." And that is as it should be, no doubt.

Still . . . you worry.

There is nothing wrong with worrying about old Hector. You would be remiss if you didn't. He lives in a world you made, and so far as he can comprehend you operate it solely for your pleasure and his benefit. You are responsible for his well-being, and a continuing, foresighted concern is an excellent preventive and good medicine for any condition. I mean sensible worry. An informed and purposeful awareness. Not frantic hand wringing. Not visions of lurking catastrophes and lingering ills unknown in the annals. That sort of worry is not only useless. It is destructive.

I have known people—as you have—who were capable

of building up enough fright-wig fear of the future to keep both them and their dogs from enjoying what could have been years of relaxed pleasure. Some get the vigils as soon as old Hector is off his feed for a day. If they have to bring the dog to the veterinarian's office with some minor complaint, they come with countenances that would cast gloom over a lively wake. They seem to have been born dejected, and they remain unshakably convinced that the worst is yet to come. Nothing cheers them. Their dogs can be treated, but the owners themselves remain resolutely disconsolate.

There are dozens of ways to worry frivolously and foolishly. The most likely way, I suppose, is to begin to think of the old dog as a person. For some people that's easy. Almost unavoidable, it seems. By the time he is old, Hector has become everything a dog can be—a pleasure, a comfort, a companion. And more. Of all friends he is the most reliable, the least demanding, the most undeviating. And with only another short step he has become a person. It happens. Often.

People dogs are, of course, remarkably like their owners, and it is not surprising that they are invariably endowed with the same feelings. I have clients whose dogs always wear booties when the weather turns nippy simply because the circulation in their owners' extremities has slowed down. It is not unusual for an owner to refuse to let me perform a simple life-saving operation because he has a phobic fear of what such people always call "the knife." Some years ago I got myself charmed into a situation in which I had to make weekly house calls to give a little old dog injections—because her mistress had never ventured into an automobile and refused even to think of sending her dog out in one of those contraptions. I once asked the dowager if she was not concerned about the dangers *I* faced in driving to her house.

"My dear boy," she said, "I pray for you."

But sometimes worry compounds fear and distorts it.

Or turns it inside out. I remember a man who once brought in a dog with an enormous tumor bulging on his side—a common enough growth, but the largest I had ever seen. When I asked the man why he hadn't done something about it sooner, he hemmed around. "Well . . . it didn't seem much when I first noticed it—last year, I guess. I couldn't see that it hurt him much, and he's getting so old. . . ." *All* of the wrong answers.

"And now he's still older," I said. "And with a tumor that size—what am I supposed to do now?"

"Well, if it turns out to be too big . . . maybe . . . I thought you could just give him a little more anesthetic. . . ."

The man's mumbling callousness infuriated me, and I determined to save that little old dog if there was any conceivable way to do it. And save him we did. With the whole staff in attendance. When the man came to take his dog home, I watched him with what I certainly hoped was a baleful eye. I remember wondering, with much less than Christian charity whether I had done either the dog or the man a favor. And whether *he* thought it a favor.

I was wrong about the man. He wasn't mean. And he wasn't callous. He was frightened. For days after the operation he called to reassure me. "He's fine today, Doc, fine. Just fine. I couldn't believe . . ." And he brought the dog in two or three times later for "little things that ought to be fixed."

The last time I heard from the man he called to say that he wouldn't be seeing us anymore. And once again I misunderstood him. I thought he meant that the old dog had died, and I began to say that I was sorry. But that wasn't it. He just wanted to tell us he was moving out of town. And he did. With a very old dog and all of his records from our files.

Your concern for your old dog—every owner's concern—is to some extent tinged with fear. Understandably so. You can't ignore the fact that there *are* severe and debilitating diseases and that some dogs do contract them. Nobody suggests that you should close your mind and eyes to real dangers. On the contrary, you should know what they are. You should be alert to their early signs. You should be prompt in reporting them to your veterinarian. But you should also realize that the major ills that owners worry about most are neither as common nor as catastrophic as most people think. You should know that at least half of the diseases that were once so devastating can now be prevented or cured or controlled, that the recent and spectacular medical discoveries that have benefited you are also used routinely today in the treatment of your dog. Far too many owners continue to live with frightful specters simply because their concept of veterinary medicine is a good half-century out of date.

Another difficulty is that our memories and perceptions are both notoriously perverse and selective. It is no effort at all to recall the details of the trouble the mailman's brother had with his old dog. But who notices that half of the good dogs he sees on the street have graying muzzles? Or thinks that it is in the least surprising that he is bowled over again by the enthusiastic fourteen-year-old dog who greets him at his neighbor's door?

Among my patients there are scores of old dogs—aged animals, fourteen- and sixteen-year-olds, and some nearly twenty. I see a great deal of them, not often enough (generally) when they are well, and much more frequently when they aren't. I can assure you that they are not weary and slow of foot. Some are amiable. Some are solemnly dignified. Some are crotchety. And one is a clown —really—who at the snap of a finger is anxious to start the routine that brought the house down in the old days. There are those among them who have their problems, of course. But whatever their difficulties, they bear them lightly—or stoically—and well. None of them needs sympathy. Nor do their owners.

It is unfair to old dogs, I think, to say only that they

generally remain active and alert. They often improve with age. And far from becoming a problem for his owner, many a seasoned and devoted old fellow has become an important sustaining presence in the house. Everybody remembers some lonely person who would have been lost without the companionship of his dog. For old people especially, dogs often provide a needed center of interest and an incentive for activity. During the last few years there has been much talk about studies that indicate that the presence of any living thing can stimulate activity in those who have lost interest in life—plants used in hospital therapy, birds in prison cells. Not everybody was surprised to learn that life sparks life. Dogs have been serving that purpose nobly for centuries.

Old dogs have often been therapeutic in small ways that merit no more, perhaps, than footnotes in the literature. A number of years ago I had a client, a middle-aged scholarly man, who had a Beagle of sorts. The man was always somewhat withdrawn, but when his wife died suddenly, he became almost a recluse. I was told that he rarely left the house and that he had even given his old Beagle to a son who lived in another city.

I didn't see the man for a long time, but one day he appeared at the office to ask advice about shipping an old dog by plane. With some prodding he yielded a little more information about his problem. He had consulted his doctor about the severe and persistent headaches he had been having, and when it appeared that they might be caused by some unusual eye condition, he had been bucked up the medical line until he came at last to the ultimate professorial specialist. The professor put him through a series of impressively scientific tests, and when they proved to be inconclusive, spent considerable time interrogating his patient. "Ah so," the doctor said, summing up the conversation. "Ah so. . . . You read very much. You research. You sit at your desk. You write your paper. You research some more. Nothing else. So . . . I will give you a prescription." And he did. My friend looked at it and protested, but the professor dismissed him imperiously." "You have my prescription," he said.

"I thought you might be interested in the prescription—as a veterinarian," the man said, handing it to me. It read: "Rx. One small dog. Walk one half hour, three times per day."

The professor was right. My friend got his old Beagle back and the headaches did disappear.

Until recently there was almost no systematic study of the aging process in dogs—or in other animals, for that matter. What we knew was minimal and doubtful. What we thought and felt was largely the reflection of traditional wisdom and of our own casual and haphazard observations. And neither was very dependable or useful. But in the last few decades we have at last begun to assemble reliable information in a purposeful fashion. We still need to learn much more, it is true. But certainly we know incomparably more than we did only a few years ago.

I say that *we* know and *we* are learning. By that I mean that researchers and scientists—and since we are talking here about dogs—veterinarians know. I wish I could tell you that the material is in the hands of those most concerned—the owners of old dogs. I wish I could say that much sound and useful information is available to you—or even that with diligent effort you could find it somewhere in some kind of understandable form. I can't. It is scattered and elusive. In veterinary medicine text after text is published on almost every aspect of health and disease—except those specifically related to aging. In some of those excellent books you may be able to find here and there a mention of age and its effects—dangling, usually, at the end of a long technical discussion: "In older dogs the results indicate . . ." Now and then an article on a new way of treating one of the degenerative diseases appears in a professional journal. And if you know what you are looking for—and where to look—you may discover it somewhere, graphed and filed away in a research paper. Even for the veterinarian it is difficult to find what he must have. For the layman to assemble what he wants and needs is next to impossible.

There is an appalling lack of readable, available material. I haven't even been able to provide a respectable list of worthwhile reading for my own clients. And many of them have asked. Some, I find, have taken to studying articles on related diseases in human beings when they want more detailed information about problems their dogs have. I don't object to that. Indeed, I encourage owners to do as much research as they can, for the information they gather generally serves as a basis for an easy, productive discussion of the dog's difficulties. Usually there is no trouble in reaching an understanding about the critical differences between man and beast. But occasionally there have been problems. Strangely, it seems that doctors—and sometimes doctors' wives—are the ones most likely to make unwise and unwarranted assumptions. I now suggest that as a professional courtesy they call me before they treat their dogs, and I have a standing agreement with my surgeon friends that I will not operate on their patients if they won't operate on mine.

As their dogs grow older owners feel an increasing sense of responsibility. Thoughtful owners—those who are most deeply concerned with keeping their dogs healthy and happy—feel that they have a special problem. And they do. It is not whether they *can* or *will* be able to cope with the difficulties that may arise. Of course they can. And of course they will. They couldn't imagine doing anything else. But more than that, they want to do everything they can to prevent and minimize those difficulties. They want to know what they can and should do to make it easy for the old dog to live out his years happily and comfortably. Their problem is in learning *how* to cope—and how to cope *well.*

And that, I suppose, is your problem too.

If it is, and if you are like my clients, you have questions. Certainly they do. They are not nervous people, most of them. They are not unduly alarmed about that unforeseeable future. And certainly they don't feel overwhelmed by their responsibilities. But they are deeply concerned. And they do ask questions. Insistently. Relentlessly, it sometimes seems.

What are the first signs of aging?
How rapidly does aging progress?
What can be done to slow it down?
Do all old dogs get degenerative diseases?
Are they always progressive?
How painful are they?
How can you tell how much pain he has?
Do old dogs know they are old?
Can an old dog be operated on?
Must he still get shots?
Can an old dog be prevented from gaining weight?
Do old dogs often become senile? When?
Should my old dog get more exercise? Or less?
Does he need vitamins and supplements?
Should he have a special diet?
Do old dogs have heart attacks? Strokes?
. . . and they go on.

There are answers to those questions. They are not always short and easy. Nor are they as neat and mathematically precise as we would like them to be. Often—generally—they have to be modified or qualified to fit the circumstances.

But there *are* answers—practical, understandable answers that should help you solve your problem. And Hector's, too.

Some of them—most of them, I hope—you will find in the discussions that follow.

II
Who Is an Old Dog?

Nobody knows how many dogs there are in the United States, much less how many old dogs there are. The figures we use are all guesses—or, if you prefer your inaccuracy by another name, estimates. And you have to go a long way around to arrive at the shaky numbers we do have.

The United States Bureau of the Census reported that as of April 1, 1970, there were 51,168,599 families in the United States. (You should always start with at least one indisputable fact, I think. Everybody believes the Census Bureau when it announces vast totals. It is only when it gets down to little numbers—the population of the town where you live, for example—that people begin to question the findings.) Tests and samplings that have been made from time to time, mostly for commercial purposes, have shown on average that two-thirds of all families have a dog. Or more than one. That would indicate that there are 35 million dogs among us. Which is almost certainly an underestimate. If you make corrections for the families that were missed in the census, the many-dog families, the dogs owned by people who are not statistically families, the dogs who are not owned by anyone, and if you add even a modest number to allow for the obvious increase in the percentage of people who are keeping dogs in recent years, you will have to raise that estimated total substantially. Make it a conservative 40 million.

Now you have a place to begin. If there are 40 million dogs of all ages, how many *old* dogs are there? And here we have nothing better than another guess. For years it has been said—and generally accepted, I think—that the average dog lives to be about eleven years old. That figure was based on common experience and observation and was probably as accurate as any of the others we have. But within the last decade or so, because of broad advances in veterinary medicine and a general increase in concern for the welfare of dogs, the life span has been considerably extended, particularly in the upper range. There are more old dogs today, and they live longer than they used to. I am talking about adult, cared-for dogs now, you must remember. If the figures were to include the outrageous number of stray and unwanted dogs who die unnoticed or are deliberately destroyed and newborn puppies with their high mortality rate, the conclusions would be vastly different. But here we are considering your kind of dog, the kind that has a responsible owner and gets decent care. It is reasonable, I think, to assume that such dogs have an average life expectancy of twelve years.

But still we haven't decided what an old dog is or when he becomes old. If you are to judge by behavior, which is the sensible way, there is no answer which is right or even acceptable. The pattern of aging varies too widely and too unpredictably. But, allowing for the great variations which do occur, if you measure in years as most people do, it seems reasonable to think of a ten-year-old as an old dog. Once again, nobody knows how many such dogs there are, but certainly there are an enormous number of them. Any veterinarian—and almost anybody else who works with or around dogs, I think—will tell you that at least 20 or 25 percent of those they see are ten years old or more. That, figure, applied to our 40 million all-dog estimate, indicates that there is an astonishing total of 8 or 10 million old dogs abroad in the land. And I believe it. For round-figure comfort and convenience (and to escape from this thicket of estimates) I am willing to accept that figure until some enterprising canine statistician can provide a more persuasive one.

Doubtful and imprecise as these estimates are, I think they should be significant to you. If we are living with that many old dogs, then clearly there must be a vast number of people who have the same problems that you have. For whatever comfort there may be in that. Frankly, I think you should find considerable encouragement in that thought, for certainly all those people out there aren't being overwhelmed by dog difficulties. More important, the figures should indicate to you that all those old dogs are not having the pangs and pains that many apprehensive owners expect them to have. For your own peace of mind I think you should abandon as quickly as you can the too prevalent idea that old dogs usually become dependent invalids. They don't. They are out there on the street with the other dogs you see. They aren't limping along in pain, they haven't gone into a disastrous decline, and they haven't become a burden to themselves or their owners. They have adjusted to the problems of aging remarkably well. They are still good dogs and good companions. Their health is dependably good and their spirits are as high (often higher these days, I think) as those of their owners. If they are less active than they once were, they are more tractable—a change which their owners are glad to attribute to their long-delayed success in training them. Many owners happily report that their old dogs are better companions and a greater pleasure to have around the house than they ever were when they were younger.

I am not trying to persuade you that for a dog old age is golden. For dogs, as for people, old age is not always a pleasure. But it is perverse and destructive for an owner to think of the dog's old age as a looming, unavoidable affliction. It need not be. With the kind of care the dog deserves (and can get today), it is just as likely to turn out to be a surprisingly easy and untroubled time.

Dogs do grow old. And they are vulnerable to the ills that are commonly associated with old age. But the aging process does not generally begin as early as most owners expect, nor is the decline as precipitous. On the contrary, the early signs of aging are likely to be so slight and to progress so slowly that for a long time they go unnoticed. Nevertheless, and for reasons which I have never been able to fathom, I find that a surprising number of owners seem to think that a representative graph of a dog's life would look somewhat like a pyramid with the tip lopped off—

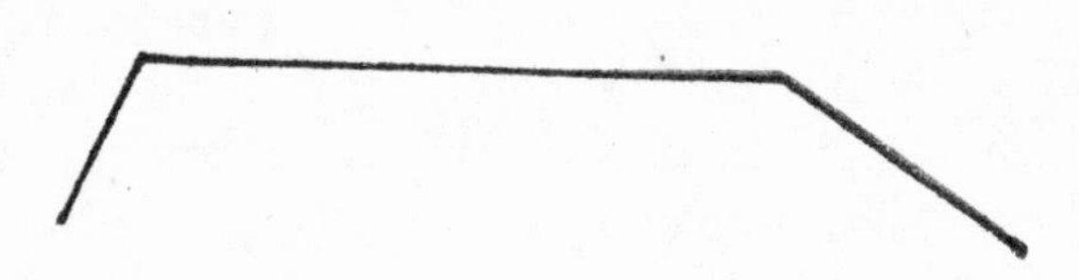

—a sharp rise from birth to maturity, a brief leveling off in secure good health, and then, inevitably, a steep and rapid decline into the difficulties of old age and senility.

Dogs don't, of course, live that sort of angular up-and-down existence. If you were to draw a graph that more accurately reflected the physical stages of a dog's life, it would probably look something like this:

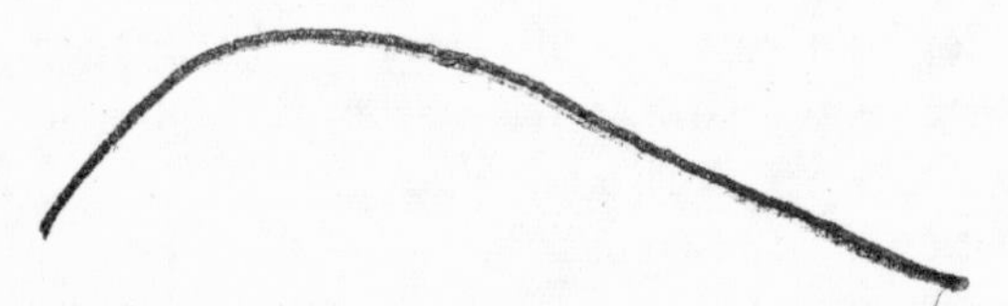

—a smooth line with no acute dramatic angles at all and a relatively slow and gradual decline into old age. A curve of this sort reflects what you might find if you were to plot the histories of a thousand dogs. It is not a prediction. Within the group there could be—and certainly would be—individual variations from the expected norm. I suppose that it is these occasional and unpredictable expectations which owners hear about that sometimes cause them to become overly concerned about the problems their own dogs may encounter as they grow older.

There are not many general rules about aging that you can depend on. One of the few that you should remember, I think, is this: If it seems to you that your dog has begun to age suddenly and if the progress appears to be rapid, you can be reasonably sure that the problem is not age itself. It is a disease or a pathological condition of some sort that is causing the change in the dog. Don't assume that he is merely showing the signs of his age. And, above all, don't wait to see what happens. Report the symptoms to your veterinarian and give him the chance to correct the condition before it reaches the point of no return.

There are always a few people who, in spite of all the evidence to the contrary, persist in thinking that their dogs are aging early and fast. They count the calendar and they think, as they say, that the dog should act his age. In fact, they insist on it. They seem to think that a dog who remains too active is recklessly squandering the energy he was endowed with, and to prevent him from coming to an early end they are prepared to hustle him into a premature retirement.

Many years ago, I remember, a woman—the kind we used to call a dear old lady—came to my office with her big, boisterous Boxer. Both were aging, but the dog still displayed a great deal of strength and energy which the wispy old lady no longer had. There was a reason for this odd mismatch, I found out. The dog had been a gift from a favorite grandson, but whether the boy was a prankster or the dog was a planned attempt to inject new activity into the lady's bland life, I never knew.

The woman was greatly concerned about the dog's health, but on examination I found nothing of any consequence wrong with him. But his mistress felt that he was getting old and that his activities should be restricted and controlled. I couldn't help her much with that. Though she had a perfectly safe fenced yard, she insisted on walking the dog sedately on a leash. I pointed out that though it might be comic-book fun to see a boy being towed through the snow by a husky dog in pursuit of a neighbor's cat, it might be calamitous instead of laughable if she found herself in a similar situation. But she could neither be advised nor frightened. She continued to worry about the dog, and I kept on worrying about her. Needlessly so, for she walked the dog without accident until she became housebound.

But there are always the ironies. When the old lady could no longer take care of the dog, he was returned to the grandson who, as it happened, did not have a secure yard and was forced to leash-walk the dog. Sure enough, one icy day. . . . I saw the boy sometime later with the cast still on his arm. It wasn't a bad break, he said. And it wasn't a cat the dog was chasing. It was another dog.

A too early and too eager concern about aging is not a major sin. From the veterinarian's point of view it is more amusing than distressing, and though the dogs may chafe a bit under capricious restrictions, it would take an extraordinary effort for an owner to impose restraints severe enough to cause serious damage. But overprotectiveness can be a source of useless worry. What begins as a small foolishness in time often becomes a burden. And burdened owners are bad owners.

Everybody has the same questions. Everybody wants to know what is going to happen as his dog grows older. As you have seen, there are averages and statistics. But a dog is not an average. He is insistently individual. There are as-a-rule generalities aplenty—and every one of them is riddled with exceptions. The only thing that you can be sure of is that your dog will do his best to exceed the average and with the help that you can give him he has as good a chance as any dog of becoming a special exception.

I am surprised at the number of exceptions that I find in my own practice. If, as we assume, dogs normally live to be about twelve years old, you might reasonably expect that by the time they were nine or ten most of them would begin to show signs of wear. And yet, though I would guess that half of those I see are that old, the majority of them have not developed difficulties that can be attributed to their age. Plainly they are no longer pups, but on the whole they are sturdy, active animals with no apparent inclination to retreat to a quiet corner. A good number of them reach twelve or more before they have any real disabilities, and when they are able to get that far without straining they have an excellent chance to keep right on going until they become canine Methuselahs.

Few dogs, I think, reach an age that would make them canine counterparts of human centenarians. And it is difficult to say what that would be in calendar years. The old method for converting dog-years to man-years, and the one that is most commonly used today, I think, is to multiply the dog's age by seven—a system that is both simple and preposterously wrong. A dog who is a year old has none of the attributes of a seven-year-old child, nor is a dog a preadolescent when he is nearing two. He may be middle-aged when he is seven, but it is ridiculous to think that a fourteen-year-old dog will have the characteristics of an old gentleman nearing one hundred.

There is no meaningful way to equate the ages of dog and man, but I can suggest a method that may be a bit more plausible. Think of the dog's first year as the equivalent of twenty-one years for a person, and then add four for every dog-year thereafter. Thus:

$$
\begin{aligned}
\text{A 3-year-old dog} &= 21 + (2 \times 4) = \text{29-year-old man} \\
\text{7-year-old dog} &= 21 + (6 \times 4) = \text{45-year-old man} \\
\text{14-year-old dog} &= 21 + (13 \times 4) = \text{73-year-old man} \\
\text{20-year-old dog} &= 21 + (19 \times 4) = \text{97-year-old man}
\end{aligned}
$$

The giant breeds—and perhaps a few others—are generally not as long-lived as the all-dog average. For them it would be more realistic to add seven for each year after the first. For example, if you were counting years for an outsized dog, you would calculate:

$$\text{A 7-year-old dog} = 21 + (6 \times 7) = \text{63-year-old man}$$

This table may not be *right,* but it is not utterly ridiculous.

Rarely do I see a dog who is authentically twenty. I do know a good many owners who tell me that their dogs are that old, but usually they are people who clearly remember that they got the pup the year the barn burned down and that was . . . let's see now. . . . One veteran that I remember well was a verifiable twenty. The card that was made out when he first arrived at my office shows that he was there for his first "puppy shots" and describes him as a mongrel Terrier. The last entry, made when he came in for a routine checkup shortly after his twentieth birthday, notes that his teeth were in excellent shape, that there was very little graying in the black markings of his face, that he showed no symptoms of the common degenerative diseases. On the final card, I noticed that the office wit had typed the name in capitals and underlined it in red. JUNIOR, it read. Later that summer he died suddenly at his owner's vacation place, apparently of a stroke.

It must be said, however, that there are exceptions at the other end of the spectrum too. I remember just as clearly the puzzling and frustrating case of a black Cocker Spaniel some years ago. Young dogs of most breeds rarely have dental problems, but he began to have trouble with his teeth before he was fully mature and before he was four he had lost most of them. By that time, too, his muzzle had grayed and then turned white. We at first suspected a hormonal deficiency but we were unable to discover any by tests. While we were still searching for clues, the dog developed a heart problem which with some difficulty we were able to control. But not long after that we discovered the beginning of a chronic kidney ailment, and in spite of early and intensive treatment, he died before his fifth birthday.

Neither of these cases is unusual. Similar instances turn up in every veterinarian's office, and for the most part they remain unexplained. These unexpected departures from the norms occur at random, and why they happen and what causes them we do not know. Veterinarians have learned a great deal about the aging process in general, and they are able to control and alleviate many of the difficulties associated with it. But still they do not know what triggers it and why there should be such wide variations in the time of its onset and in the rate at which it progresses.

It is well known, of course, that many factors in one way or another affect the general health and longevity of a dog. Their effects have been studied for years, and they are being even more thoroughly explored now. But most of them are believed to be peripheral, contributing factors rather than primary causes. Nutrition undoubtedly plays an important part. Proper medical care, or the lack of it, can and does make a measurable difference. The lingering and debilitating effects of early disease have long been recognized as a significant element in the background. But none of these factors in themselves nor all of them together adequately explain the variations which exist.

It has become increasingly evident, I believe, that the ultimate explanation for these differences will be found in the genetic heritage which a dog carries. Every dog, from the moment he becomes a fertilized ovum, bears his own unique genetic imprint. And most researchers now believe that it is primarily this indelible design which sets the unchanging and unchangeable pattern of his development.

That is not to say, of course, that every dog is predestined to reach a certain age and that nothing will change his fate. It does suggest, however, that the outer limits of his life are determined by the genes he carries and there is no evidence that anything can be done to alter that fact. But implicit in that concept there is also the belief that if he can be helped to escape the quirks and hazards of accident and disease, he can and should reach his full programmed potential.

If the secrets of aging and longevity are locked in his genes, you have little hope of predicting with any accuracy the particular pattern that your dog will follow as he grows older. You can't examine his genes, and there is no way for you to discover whether he is programmed for eight or ten years or for twice that number. You can't know that when he is eight he will be in his complacent middle age and that old age will still be far in the future. He runs on his own inward chronology. Calendars and birthdays mean much less to him than they do to you. Most of what you want to know about his future you will have to learn from the changes you see as they actually occur. Your only reliable guide is observation. Prophecy is useless.

What are these changes likely to be? What are the signs by which you will recognize them?

The earliest signs are subtle and obscure, so slight and day-to-day gradual that they are almost certain to go unnoticed at the time. But later you may remember them as the first indications of aging. There are small behavioral changes. Among the first is a slow decline in exuberance, in inquisitiveness, in the need for busyness and commotion, particularly in the small bouncing breeds. A few common changes in physical appearance occur about the same time, and though they vary from breed to breed and appear in random sequence, you can expect them in due course. There will be a little graying around the muzzle —only a slight rinsed look with the blonds but a rather rakish touch with the darker types. The coat will grow a little more slowly than it once did and it will not be quite so luxuriant. In the wintertime it will not be quite as lustrous and in the spring the shedded hair will be less abundant on the furniture. You will notice that sometimes Hector will be quite satisfied to end the fetch-the-ball game before your arm is tired, and the next day he may move as though he has the same slight discomfort that you feel in your back and legs after you have spent a weekend mowing and raking.

His eating and drinking habits will change, too. He will probably take more fluids, and you will notice that his relief trips are more urgent and frequent. At mealtime he will be less ravenous than he used to be, inclined to pick out the best bits first, to expect more generous garnishes of table scraps, to leave his pan unlicked and unpolished. He doesn't require as much food because he has begun to be less active and needs less to sustain himself. If you are an easy touch, if you continue to give him as much of his regular food as he had in the past (enhanced now with added tasty morsels), you'll soon have another sign of aging. He will begin to put on weight. And that is more than a sign. It is a problem. But more of that elsewhere.

Both Penelope and Hector will begin to be less concerned with matters sexual. She will be in heat less frequently, perhaps, and less urgently. Hector will no longer hustle about sprinkling so industriously, nor will he find it necessary to range so far from the house to find trees and bushes suitable for the purpose. His testicles will become somewhat smaller, and though he will not be oblivious to feminine charm, he will not find every bitch on the block irresistibly attractive.

In time these and other physical changes will become more apparent. His muzzle will become noticeably gray, sometimes quite white. His teeth, always one of his strong points, may begin to loosen slightly, and because of infections around the gums or on his lips, he may for the first time develop a socially offensive halitosis. When he is lying down, he will wait for a sufficient reason to get up, take his time to stretch more thoroughly, and when he does move off, it will take a little distance for him to limber up and get the stiffness out of his joints. Because he will be covering much less mileage, his nails will grow long and, particularly if he isn't free to spend much time on abrasive outdoor footing, you will have to trim them both to keep him comfortable and to reduce the clatter on bare floors. And sometime, while all this is going on, you will start to worry when you notice that the pupils of his eyes seem to be a bit clouded and turning a milky gray. Although they are, you needn't be alarmed about cataracts. It is a normal change and it occurs in all dogs as they grow older.

During this time there is a parallel, but much less evident, slowing of the reflexes and a decline in the sharpness of the senses. But it is so gradual that you may be unaware of the change for a long time. Hector will compensate so well that you can easily fail to realize he is having difficulties with sight and sound.

With working dogs—hunting dogs, for example—the changes are more noticeable. And, as every hunter knows, the results are not all bad. The overenthusiastic dog quiets down and learns to work more efficiently. He is forced to depend more on his nose, and the scenting ability seems to be the one sense that is not dulled by age. If his hearing is less acute, he will be more intent on following where his nose leads and less likely to be distracted by the baying of the hounds off in some other direction. If he doesn't see well, he will not be tempted to leave the trail and take the shortcut to the opposite hill. This midcareer doesn't last forever, of course, and sooner or later the seasoned old hunter is unable to keep up with his young rivals. But while these interim years last, the old boy may well be the most reliable dog in the field.

The beginning of the aging process—if, indeed, it can properly be called a *beginning* since, as with all living things, it actually starts at birth—often amounts to little more than a slowing down of all of the processes of the body. As he grows older, the dog sheds his need for restless, compulsive activity and appears content to cruise along conservatively and comfortably. He seems to be untroubled by the changes that are occurring, or, at most, to be only mildly inconvenienced by them.

With good care, good genes, and a good constitution a dog usually weathers the onset of age with only slight discomforts and few, if any, real difficulties. But though there are no obvious signs of failing, the aging process is continuing. The machine simply doesn't function as efficiently as it once did. Gradually it begins to show evidence of wear. It runs down. It is no longer able to repair and rebuild and replenish as quickly and easily as it once did. Local, minor, and temporary malfunctions begin to occur with greater frequency, and though they can often be easily treated and controlled, they do have a cumulative effect on the whole system. And eventually, somewhere and sometime, there is a major breakdown—sometimes a sudden, disastrous incident such as a cerebral hemorrhage or a cardiac arrest, sometimes a concealed event like the runaway growth of an internal cancer that has outgrown its blood supply.

Often—indeed, more often than not, I think—it is difficult even for a veterinarian to say what it is that throws the machine out of kilter, what organ is directly responsible for the sequence of failure. If the dog has had regular and thorough examinations, there is a record to guide the veterinarian and he may be able to trace the difficulty to a particular organ or system that was known to be weak. But without that history, he is likely to be hard pressed to identify the triggering cause. The parts of the machine are themselves so complex and they are so delicately balanced and interrelated that it becomes immensely difficult to determine in a chain of events what is cause and what is effect.

Think for a moment of one common sequence. Hector is well along in years. He has had no history of illness and no special problems have been identified, so we must assume that all of the organs and all of the systems of his body have been about equally stressed. They are all in working order, but all of them have been weakened and worn by time so that though the whole machine continues to function, it is operating with decreased efficiency. It is vulnerable to a disrupting accident in any part. One day Hector is getting along as well as usual in his staid, relaxed fashion. But the next day, let us suppose, he makes the mistake of eating something that doesn't agree with him. It needn't be something toxic or outrageously indigestible. It can be anything—even too much of a perfectly innocuous substance—which disturbs his digestive process. But it is sufficient to create an uncommon stress on his digestive system. That, in turn, puts an increased burden on his kidneys to eliminate the extra waste material. If they are unable to increase their activity enough or do the job thoroughly enough, there is a buildup of toxins in the bloodstream. There are then heavier demands on the heart to circulate more blood to the lungs and the kidneys in order to cleanse it more rapidly. And if the worn old heart is unable adequately to meet those demands, Hector becomes another victim of congestive heart failure. Or so we say. Actually it was the failure of the whole interdependent mechanism, the ultimate though unpredictable collapse of the one-hoss shay.

But the shay doesn't always collapse in a heap. Repairs are often possible. Perhaps the incident was triggered by a known weakness in one organ or one system of the dog's body—his kidneys, for example. If the rest of his body is able to sustain the stress for a time, it may be quite possible to provide treatment which will reestablish the balance. Some chronic kidney diseases can be controlled with diet and medication which reduce the amount of work required of the kidneys and make it possible for them to continue to keep the blood and tissues in functional condition. Achieving this new accommodation may take time and careful adjustment, and while the treatment is going on, it may be necessary also to support the action of the heart and other organs. But if Hector can be helped through this first acute episode and his condition stabilized, there is an excellent chance that his body will be able to make the necessary adjustments. With good care and stern dietary restrictions there is no reason why he can't live comfortably and reach a respectable age.

What I have been saying about aging in dogs comes down to this:

Old age for a dog is not the ordeal that many people imagine it is. Not for the dog and not for his owner. We have in recent years greatly increased our knowledge of the processes of aging and improved our ability to cope with the problems that do arise. But even though we are able to describe with reasonable accuracy the changes that normally occur in dogs—in all dogs, as a group—the information we have is of doubtful use in predicting the effects that aging will have on any particular dog. Each is an individual and much of what happens within him as he grows older is (we think) directed and controlled by the genetic imprint with which he was born.

You can and should be guided by the knowledge and accumulated experience of those who have studied thousands of dogs. But you cannot assume that your own dog will conform to the general pattern, the average. He is likely to follow the graph in only a very general way.

If you want to know how age will affect *your* dog, what changes he will go through, what you should do now and in the future to make his old age secure and comfortable, then the best, the easiest, the most rewarding way to begin is to spend a little time finding out what the dog is right now. What you will learn by observing the dog himself will be of much more use to you than anything you can find out about what *generally* happens to *most* dogs.

III
How Much Do You Know About Hector?

A few of my best friends are doctors. M.D.s, that is. And they used to tell me that they were often stunned to discover how little their patients knew about their own bodies. If I can believe what the doctors tell me—and I did and do—the teaching of human anatomy (if there is any meaningful instruction at all) must be one of the most appalling failures of the century.

I say the doctors *used* to tell me. I am not, I'm afraid, a compulsive listener, and after hearing a few of the physicians' shockers, I often felt compelled to share with them some owner's explanation of what he thought was wrong with his dog. That turned out badly. My owners were almost invariably more confused about ailments and anatomy than the doctors' patients, and in time I found it advisable to give up that particular kind of one-upmanship.

I wouldn't want you to misunderstand the tenor of this light, after-hours medical conversation. We were not equating people and dogs. I am convinced that a decent understanding of the workings of his own body may be the most valuable knowledge that a person can acquire, far more important than knowing what makes a dog tick.

And furthermore, I wouldn't want you to read into this any implication that all patients and all owners are invincibly misinformed about themselves or their dogs.

But still, you wouldn't believe . . .

For young veterinarians just beginning to practice—for the good ones, the sharp and dedicated ones—it is a discouraging experience. When one of them comes to work with us at the hospital, I make it a practice to tell him that I expect it will take him a year to learn to keep his eyebrows in place. And it does.

"What do you mean, tonsillitis?" says the registered nurse who is not going to be taken for a fool. "Dogs don't have tonsils!"

"Microscope or no microscope, it stands to reason he ain't got worms," Old Timer argues. "I've been giving him garlic every week."

"Well, maybe I still do make some mistakes," the owner-turned-breeder admits modestly. "But one thing I know for sure. They've got to have fresh meat."

The young musician is positive. "She *can't* be pregnant! I kept her in the whole time. She and her brother Charlie. The whole time."

And the literary gentleman is astonished. "I can't believe it. He barked so much I just *assumed* he wouldn't bite."

"Yes . . . yes, she eats good," says the fat man with the fat dog. "But she gets her vitamins regular. Keeps up her strength. Prevents colds."

"Well, I never!" says the old lady indignantly, sweeping up her feeble little old dog. "Give her milk?" And as the door slams, she shouts to the world, "Milk! Milk causes worms!"

Mrs. Elegant sighs, "I really don't care, Doctor. Find a home for her someplace. We got her just to raise pups. But now that she has had those mongrels, she'll never be able to have purebred pups."

Careful Eater is proud. "Don't bother to look at his

teeth, Doc. He never had a piece of candy in his life. No sweets."

"He must *still* have worms something awful," says Worried, returning the dog with still another specimen. "I see him eating grass every day."

I have no idea how much help and hope Dr. Reuben's book *Everything You Always Wanted to Know About Sex* *

* *and were afraid to ask*

has given his readers. But I suppose that the inspired ad man who conceived the * line has been responsible for more titles without books than any person in history. The one that I won't get around to writing is, of course, *Everything You Should Know About Dogs* *

* *and would know if you'd ask your veterinarian.*

It would be a primer, of course. And for that reason, hard to do. But it is needed.

Owners, I have found, are quick to take offense when doubt is cast on their knowledge or the reliability of their opinions—and particularly ludicrous opinions—about what a dog wants and needs, or about what he must, may, or should have. And readers, I suppose, are as sensitive. But nobody, I hope, will stop reading here and go away, mistaking a wry smile for a frivolous attitude. Nobody knows enough to be snide or supercilious in a world in which what we know is only a speck on what remains to be discovered. And that is as true of veterinarians and their knowledge as it is of anybody and anything else.

This is a sad and serious matter to me, this common lack of even the basic facts about the way a dog's body is put together and the way it works. We have learned much about how to prevent, treat, and cure the great scourges which used to destroy dogs by the millions. But we still haven't been able to persuade enough owners to make the small effort it takes to learn the simple facts about how and why a dog's body functions the way it does. I am persuaded—and after thirty years in practice, I am stone-faced serious about this—that one of the great threats to dogs today is simply the lack of knowledge on the part of their owners. What owners don't know, don't notice, don't understand, kills thousands of strong dogs every year.

And if the last paragraph or so seems to have risen to an evangelical pitch, you can assume that in this matter I *am* evangelical. Militantly so.

This is a book about middle-aged dogs and old dogs, and there is enough to be said about them without attempting a refresher course on all aspects of dog care. But dogs are young before they are old, and all that any of us can learn about them is little enough. If you don't already have a good general reference book, get one. Read it. Keep it. You'll need it.

But the question we started with was: What do you know about Hector? Or Penelope?

By now you have anticipated the answer. Too little.

And perhaps it won't surprise you, either, to hear that if you are like most owners I counsel with and wrestle with, you probably know less about Hector now than you knew about him when he was a pup. It works out that way. You'll tell me, no doubt, that when you got Hector you knew nothing about dogs—or almost nothing. And that in ten years you've learned a lot from him, that's for sure. And so you have. You have *had* to learn to cope with a dog.

But I still say it is unlikely that you know *old* Hector as well as you knew Hector when he was a pup. He was new then—cute and unpredictable and endlessly interesting. He was a puzzle. He was a problem. And he was the center of attention. He had to be. He made puddles and you wiped up—or, even worse, somebody else wiped up and reported him to you each time. He didn't eat for a whole day—and then ate too fast and regurgitated in the middle of the guest-room rug. For months, no matter what you were doing, you watched him out of the corner of your eye and rushed him outdoors the instant he got that search-and-squat look. You took him to the veterinarian for inoculations, dewormings, and checkups. You taught him to *sit* and *stay* (when there were no overpowering distractions) and to walk on the leash without choking himself or tripping you very often, to ride in the car without helping you to drive, to bark responsibly when somebody came to the door, and to subside when you greeted the intruder.

I doubt you really think that you know Hector now as well as you did then. Now he is simply *there*. He has learned the rules and adapted to the conventions of the house. His habits are well established, his needs are (you think) known and predictable, his activities have been coordinated with the family routine. He dozes more, barks less, respects the furniture, and greets the weekend dog-sitter, you are told, like a lost friend. He is a quiet, responsible member of the family who requires very little special attention. And gets exactly that.

I am not accusing anyone of neglect. Or even of a waning interest in Hector. I am merely describing what happens in most well-regulated homes—a natural and normal development. As a matter of fact, the change is, in part, Hector's own doing. He is perfectly content with the smooth way the world operates. He doesn't demand and apparently doesn't need the amount of attention he once got. Certainly he is less insistently energetic than he used to be. He still wants his walk, of course, but more to please you than to amuse himself. He's happy to go for a ride if you suggest it, but he doesn't leap into the car every time the door is opened. To him, comfort has become at least as important as excitement, and watching you work in the garden is just as satisfying as helping you to dig. By his own choice, then, Hector is *there*. Just being there is important. And to him it seems natural, comfortable, and sufficient.

It isn't sufficient, however. There is a real danger that in this complacent atmosphere Hector will recede into the wallpaper. The inclination to let sleeping dogs lie (like the compulsion to grab a cliché that was actually made for the purpose) is difficult to resist. It is easy to ignore the changes that are taking place and it is natural to assume that all those which cannot be overlooked are the normal, unavoidable, progressive signs of aging. Some of them are, of course, but it is a mistake to assume that all of them are. They may also be abnormal, entirely avoidable and progressive only if they go unnoticed and untreated. The fact that old Hector seems content and does not complain does not necessarily mean that all is well with him. It means merely that he can't or doesn't complain and that if you are to have early warning of developing difficulties, you will have to gather them from what you know and what you see.

By saying that it is common and easy to let old Hector become an unnoticed fixture, I don't mean to condone it. It is negligence—a benign negligence, perhaps, but negligence nevertheless, and often a major factor in the untimely and needless loss of a stout dog. By now, certainly, the importance of early diagnosis has become a tattered truism, and everybody who can read and cipher must know that trivial conditions can and sometimes do become disasters. You wouldn't believe that it would be necessary to remind sensible people they should have a lively enough interest in their own dogs to notice when something is beginning to go wrong. You wouldn't think so. But it is.

It is dangerous to let yourself drift into the common present-and-accounted-for attitude with your dog. When he was young, he was an under-foot presence, and when anything did go wrong, there was usually an obvious and dramatic change. But the difficulties that develop with age often creep up slowly and their symptoms are far more subtle. To discover them as promptly as you should, you'll have to do more than merely *see* the dog. You'll have to be *aware* of him. You'll have to learn to *observe* him.

It's not a great chore to keep tabs on the old boy. It is simply a matter of being reasonably conscious of the way he behaves—how he walks and runs, how quickly and surely he reacts, how he eats and drinks and sleeps and plays. It requires no effort to notice whether he hops into the car or makes it one leg at a time, whether he is at the door when you put the key in the lock or still asleep when you get in, whether *you* watch for the mailman or Hector announces his arrival, whether *he* first stops roughhousing or *you* do. It is only a matter of being conscious of what's happening and realizing that it has meaning.

And without making a white-coat-and-stethoscope event of it, you can surely find time every couple of weeks to examine him a little more carefully. Run your fingers over his body. Is his coat still smooth and healthy? Do you notice any lumps, bumps, bulges, or rough spots? Are there any areas that have been scratched red and bare? Are there any changes about his eyes or his eyelids? Is his nose clean and clear? Do you notice an offensive odor in his ears? Do his lips and gums and teeth look normal to you? Is there any change or any discharge around his genitals or body openings? Do you find *anything* unusual that you don't understand? If you are very conscientious about it, it might take you as much as three minutes to check all of these things. Does that seem excessive?

Routine observations of this sort should fall under the heading of minimal care and attention. It is hard to believe that any person could become so apathetic and unconcerned he would fail to pay even that much attention to his dog. And yet, I must tell you, I am no longer surprised when an owner looks as if he had never really seen his dog until I put him up on the table in my office. "Well, look at that, now!" he says in amazement when I uncover a growth the size of a walnut on the dog's flank. "You know, Doc, I never noticed that." I'm not surprised. I just don't know what to say.

With no effort at all you can do better. Much better.

What *should* you know about Hector? I am a most agreeable man. If anything, I am altogether too tolerant of careless owners, I think. (To the point of getting dubious compliments. An owner told me recently that she had brought her dog to me because she had been told that I was gentle—with owners.) But in my book every owner ought to have at least a certain minimal knowledge of his own dog. If you take your dog to a veterinarian, he is going to want to know a bit more about him than what he can see. He will ask you questions—specific questions intended to provide him with the background information he needs. They won't be difficult questions and they won't require specialized knowledge. If you are, by any reasonable standard, a conscientious and observant owner, you should be able to answer them accurately and sensibly.

The number of questions and the types of questions the veterinarian asks will, of course, depend on the dog's condition. It will also depend on how knowledgeably you are able to answer. If you grope and stumble about, the veterinarian won't embarrass you at length. But if you can give him meaningful answers, he may ask you many questions. Your answers will help him. And help your dog.

Here are a few questions of the sort he may ask. With an occasional note.

How old is the dog? Not: "Well . . . Dear, was it the year *after* grandfather died or . . . ?" In years. How old he is *does* make a difference.

Has he had any serious illnesses in the past? Not: "Well, some time back he didn't seem to feel so hot when . . ." Any treated, serious illnesses?

What were they? A name would be good. But symptoms and treatment will do.

How much does he weigh? Sure, he can weigh him. But do *you* know?

Has he gained or lost weight in the last year? Yes or no. Not: "It looks to me a little like . . ."

When did you last weigh him? Hm-m-m-m?

Do you think he has gained or lost three pounds in the past three months? Hard to tell, isn't it? But three pounds could be 10 or 15 percent of his weight. And that's significant.

How much do you think he should weigh? Yes, that *is* a test question. He'll tell you.

How much would you say he weighed when he was two years old? And so is this one.

What kind of food do you give him? Meat? Dry? Moist? Canned? What brand?

How much does he get? By weight. He won't expect you to know what that means in calories, though you should.

Does he eat it well? Or are you a coaxer?

Is he eating more or less recently?

Have you changed the type of food or amount of food recently?

Is it a "complete" food?

Do you supplement it? With what?

Why? This will tell him something about you *or* the dog.

Does he get treats? At the table? So will this, probably.

Is he drinking more water recently? Or less? Do you really know? Honestly?

Does he need to relieve his bladder more frequently?

Has there been any change in his bowel movements recently?

Is he constipated?

Does he tire easily? How do you mean?

Is he often stiff or lame? When?

How else has he changed in the last six months?

Has his personality changed?

Have you noticed that he sleeps much more lately?

Does he wake quickly when you call him?

Does he get up slowly? With difficulty?

Does he resent strangers? Snap at them?

Does anything else about him worry you?

Has he had anything like this before?

What did you do about it then?

Obviously, no veterinarian is going to ask all of these

questions. Or these particular questions. On the other hand, he may ask many that I haven't even mentioned. And he is virtually certain to pursue any line of questioning if it seems to throw light on the dog's condition.

I think you *should* be able to answer such questions. But I doubt that you could answer all of them. Or even most of them. And to tell you the truth, if I were you, I wouldn't feel too bad about that right now. Few owners could answer them properly. But this I *will* say: If, two or three weeks from now, you are *still* unable to answer such questions, you are not paying enough attention to your dog. Then, I think, you *should* feel bad.

And if you think I'm being too tough, remember: I am an *agreeable* veterinarian.

IV
When He's Very Old

Old dogs don't fade away. They grow older.

The illnesses of middle age can be handled in many ways. If the dog has proper and regular attention, they can often be prevented entirely. Frequently they can be so stabilized and controlled that the dog is hardly aware of them. Sometimes they can be completely and permanently cured. But the diseases which appear with very old age—the so-called degenerative diseases—cannot forever be prevented or avoided. They arrive in no predictable sequence and often for reasons which are not evident. They are generally described in terms of the organ or system affected—kidney disease, heart failure. But often they could more properly be considered localized failures of a worn, old system. They are simply the result of old age. And old age itself is incurable.

We should be able to admit, I think, that old age is not an easy time, for animals or for human beings. Though it need not be—and in a humane society would not be—a time of gnawing pain and discontent, the obvious discomforts and disabilities simply can't be concealed. The endless flow of anesthetizing euphemisms—sunset days, harvest years, golden times, senior-citizen serenity—may help hucksters peddle merchandise, but surely it is a disservice to everybody else. An attempt to provide a wider insight and understanding of the realities—and to do something about them—would be a more responsible way to deal with the problems. Or so I think. And this is as true for animals as it is for people.

Caring for an old dog can be a trying experience, and caring for a sick old dog week after week sometimes becomes deeply disturbing. But a dog's last years are not inevitably, or even usually, a time of daily worry and frustration for the owner. They do require the owner to protect the dog with increasing diligence, to provide the attention that will keep him as free as possible from pain and discomfort, to demonstrate the solicitude and compassion which the old dog deserves. These are not onerous chores. Most dogs do not become invalids. They may be feeble or quirky or somnolent, but they remain capable of getting along on their own with a little help and encouragement. Often the terminal illness itself is acute and mercifully brief. It need never be a prolonged agony. When life becomes hopeless or intolerably painful, the dog can be painlessly released from an unbearable situation. And though that decision itself is sometimes exceedingly difficult for the owner—a problem we will discuss later—it does remove the specter of a long and hopeless vigil over a dying dog.

In this situation, grace will be your chief asset. Nothing, in my opinion, will be as important to the welfare of the dog as your attitude. I know that throughout this book I have urgently advised you to rely on the skill and understanding of your veterinarian. And I still do. He can do a great deal to help you to keep the old dog comfortable, to relieve him of pain and discomfort. And that, in these final years, will be your principal concern. But taking the dog to the veterinarian will not in itself do anything for your attitude. And your attitude clearly will affect not only the kind of care which you give the dog but also the whole psychological climate in which he lives.

Everyone knows how acutely a dog responds to his owner's moods. Nearly every day I am told of some incident which convinces an owner that his dog has an uncanny perception. And a dog does have a kind of superperception. But it is not uncanny. Through the centuries the dog's survival has depended on his ability to recognize and interpret minimal clues, and today the most important ones are those which come from his master. He is acutely tuned to them, and even when his senses have been dulled by age—especially then, it sometimes seems—he still receives them loud and clear. He doesn't *think*. He *senses*. And with remarkable depth and accuracy. There can be no doubt, I think, that how well your dog fares during his declining years—and how troublesome those years are to you—is significantly affected by how you feel about the dog and about your responsibilities to him.

A person's disposition, personality, psychological bent —call it what you like—cannot be manipulated at will. There are those who are always troubled and depressed by contact with illness, infirmity, physical disability of any kind. Others, faced with the same situations, find in themselves enormous resources of kindness, helpfulness and understanding. There seems to be a tendency (and a growing tendency, I'm afraid) to accept these traits as fixed, immutable characteristics which cannot or should not be tampered with. In interpersonal relationships we are prone to assume a defensive attitude which says, in effect, "Well, that's the way I am. I can't help it." If that attitude is accepted as normal between people, it can, of course, be applied without a twinge of conscience in the case of an old dog. It is easy to say, "He upsets me. It disturbs me to see him wandering around. I can't help the way I feel." And some people do say just that.

I know that I am getting far afield, but since I am this

far out on a tangent, I'll go further. I think that a callous lack of concern for an old dog is poisonous in a family. Again and again people tell me that the real reason they keep a dog is that they think that having one is important for the children, that it influences their emotional and psychological development, teaches them to be responsible, molds character, and benefits them in other ways I had never even thought of. And I agree. (Indeed, I'm afraid I have amused many people, and offended a few, by saying that I think that a good dog—and a good veterinarian—can often do more for a mixed-up kid than a psychiatrist.) But these same people, people who extol the benefits of keeping a dog, can also be capable occasionally of committing psychological atrocities. I have had them scowl at me when I tell them that the old dog is not seriously ill but that in the future he *will* need special attention and regular treatment and have heard them, standing there in the midst of their children, blandly say, "Oh . . . Well, I don't see how we could manage that. I don't have the time [or patience], and Johnny . . . well, I know that Johnny wouldn't take care of him. Doctor, I guess you'll just have to . . ." And I know that if I *do* persuade them to take the dog home he will be neglected. What has happened to all those thoughts about instilling loyalty, kindness, responsibility? What has happened to those ideas about emotional growth and psychological insights? What is happening to the children?

I am not prepared to try to understand that kind of attitude. Or to excuse it. I think it is appallingly callous and selfish.

Is this about the care of an old dog? I think it is.

You can't prevent your old dog from getting older, but you *can* meet whatever problems there are with grace —with tolerance, kindness, and patience. There may be exceptions, but in most cases, I think, it is sheer selfish nonsense for a person to say that he is too sensitive, too subject to depression, to take care of an old dog. It is precisely the sensitive people who *do* care for their dogs responsibly. Sensitive people find it impossible to do otherwise.

A sense of humor helps, too. Dogs seldom become senile, if by senility you mean mental vagueness, a tendency to lose contact with the present and to drift off into an unreal world. But often they do become eccentric or quirky. They develop crotchets, get stubborn streaks, and sometimes appear to pleasure themselves in what seems to be plain cussedness. They become attached to quixotic routines, and when they persist in them—as they often do—there is little that you can do except tolerate them with whatever amusement you can muster.

An old Basset Hound who is a long-time patient of mine still insists on a long evening excursion though he has a congestive heart problem and for years has had to have a daily stimulant. In fair weather or foul he plows forward with great determination and absolutely refuses to turn back. Nor can he be persuaded to make sensible and convenient turns that would bring him back home before he becomes exhausted. If his companion insists on retracing their steps, he sits firmly and refuses to budge. And he is an inconvenient and uncooperative bundle to carry. Fortunately he lives with a multitudinous family. Whoever takes the old dog out must first tell another member of the family that he is leaving. Ten or fifteen minutes later the rescue squad sets out in the family car, picks up the leader and the tired old dog, and they all ride home in comfort. That has been the routine, they tell me, for several years.

Another owner tells me that he is sent to bed at 11:30 every night. For some time it has been his habit to see the eleven o'clock television news and then to prepare for bed. The dog waits patiently for the news broadcast to end, but if the set isn't turned off promptly at that time—if the owner tries surreptitiously to switch to another program—the dog sets up such a racket that he has to be exiled to the garage until the owner *is* ready to go to bed.

Not long ago a woman came to me to ask if there was anything that could be done to get her dog out of a wearisome rut. Both she and the old dog enjoyed taking long walks, but for months the dog had insisted on following one single, established route and by no amount of tugging or coaxing could she persuade him to depart from it. She had begun to feel, she said, as though she were on a treadmill or walking through a repetitive dream. And besides, it would occasionally be convenient to be able to drop a letter at the post office or to make a one-block detour to get a quart of milk at the local grocery. The small reconditioning program we devised worked intermittently but not reliably. When she leaves home with the dog, the woman still can't be sure that she will be able to mail the check to the telephone company.

There are always a few such characters, but most dogs, when they are very old, simply retreat into a world of diminishing response and activity. And we are as uncertain about the basic causes of the decline as we are about what triggers the final general aging process in people. One fairly recent theory is that as the body ages an increasing number of wayward, mutant cells are produced, and in time they become too numerous for the body to eliminate or control effectively. Hardening of the arteries plays its part. Worn and damaged cells are replaced more slowly; nerve tissue, always slow to rebuild, becomes less responsive. Each local weakness accelerates the general aging process, and in time the efficiency of the whole mechanism declines until it functions on only a minimal, maintenance level.

One by one new evidences of aging are added to the earlier ones. The muscles, particularly those of the upper leg, begin to waste away, and instead of being weary and slow, the dog shows signs of actual weakness. He is less confident in his gait, stumbles easily, and tires quickly. He is reluctant to go upstairs and afraid to come down.

The hair that was gray begins to thin out. The dog sleeps a great deal, sometimes so much that it seems he is seldom awake. But he sleeps fitfully, turning frequently to relieve the discomforts of his arthritis, perhaps, or coughing because of the lung congestion caused by a weakening heart. When he is aroused he often seems bewildered, and when he gets up he rises stiffly, often with a half-stifled groan. He may even snap testily if he is startled out of his sleep —and then wag his tail apologetically when he recognizes a familiar figure. If he stands up quickly, he may seem faint or giddy for a moment. He rarely bothers to bark, and when he does his voice is weak and rasping. In time his bones may become so brittle that they can be fractured by even a slight fall, and when they are broken, they are slow to mend. He drinks more often, has to go out more frequently, dribbles briefly by the nearest bush, and returns quickly. And now and then, of course, he doesn't make it to the door at all. That may be caused by a weakening of the sphincter muscles, which makes it impossible for him to hold out as long as he used to. But often it seems to be the expression of a don't-give-a-damn attitude, or a feeling that it just isn't worth the effort to plod around the house looking for somebody to open the door again. He is a very old party, and these are simply the infirmities that come at his age.

These difficulties don't descend on a dog all at once, of course, and some dogs escape many of them entirely. Those who have little or no pain often subside into a kind of amiable somnolence. Establishing a comfortable and convenient headquarters near the center of the household activity, they become passive observers, content to rest and to be reassured by the movement around them. Occasionally there are brief and unpredictable personality changes. One day an agreeable old dog may be testy or moody and withdrawn, and the next be as affectionate and responsive as ever. And always there are the unexplained remissions. An old fellow who has been entirely disinterested in what is going on around him may suddenly rouse himself from his lethargy and return to active duty, patrolling the garden and warning off intruders, real and imagined, who threaten to invade his territorial boundaries. And then, a few days later, for reasons as obscure as those that set off the burst of activity, he will return to his rocking-chair retirement and the seclusion of the house.

The thing that owners fear most, I think, is that the old dog will become blind and deaf. And the progressive loss of sight and hearing does often come with old age. But dogs compensate remarkably well, and it is common, I think, for owners to worry more than they should about these handicaps. Indeed, a dog's vision has to be extremely impaired before most people notice that anything is amiss at all. Owners sometimes bring their dogs to me when they first suspect that their vision is not quite as acute as it once was—and are stunned to learn that their dogs are already three-quarters blind, and probably have been for a long time. The loss is very gradual usually, and so long as the dog is in familiar surroundings, he gets about seemingly without much difficulty. Even after his sight is almost entirely gone, he confidently travels his usual rounds, apparently by memory, habit, and scent.

The same is true of deafness. Arteriosclerosis, which affects the middle ear, often causes a loss of hearing. Sometimes, for unknown reasons, the dog may become deaf in one ear while the other still functions quite normally. An owner often notices that his dog appears confused when he calls him—confused, of course, because the sound seems to him to come always from the direction of his good ear, which, like as not, is the wrong direction. Some dogs will occasionally and for no evident reason hold their heads high and howl lugubriously. It is thought that this may be caused by a ringing in the ears that is associated with developing deafness.

Deafness is usually progressive, but the dog accommodates as he does to the loss of vision, and probably more easily and more readily. Sometimes, in fact, diminished hearing turns out unexpectedly to be an advantage. I have had many people tell me that they were pleased that the old dog, who for years had been edgy and likely to set off prolonged false alarms at any hour of the night, had become a serene and sensible sleeper who never disturbed the family's rest—without realizing that he was sleeping more because he was hearing less. And a man once explained to me that his summers were much more pleasant after his dog was deaf. From puppyhood the dog had been afraid of thunder and every noisy shower had thrown him into a yelping frenzy. To make matters worse, the man's wife was terrified by lightning. Every summer was a series of thunder crises with the man's wife hiding her head under a blanket on the bed and the dog whining and scratching underneath. But after the dog became deaf, the man said, his trouble was cut in half.

When he is very old, a dog often slips very gradually into a kind of dotage. He putters around in his favorite spots, sometimes seeming a little foolish and confused, sometimes irritable and stubborn. He occupies as much of his old place and position as he can, resists unwelcome change, persists in his old routine as much and as long as his strength permits. Of what goes on in his head we know very little. So far as we can see, he seldom loses touch with reality or drifts off into hallucinations, and only very slowly does he lose his early conditioning. As the circle of his life closes in around him, he is occupied more and more with the simple biological necessities which contribute to survival. Eventually he arrives at the canine equivalent of second childhood and has to be protected and cared for accordingly.

As the dog grows old and feeble, your efforts will be limited largely to doing what you can to make life as pleasant and comfortable as you can for him. That can best be accomplished by being alert and responsive to his needs, by doing what needs to be done when it needs to be done. It is possible to try to do too much too soon. Oversolicitous people are inclined to become excessively concerned and protective. They guide the old boy around when he is perfectly happy and able to get about on his own, bundle him up against the first nip in the air, worry needlessly about his declining appetite. Aside from spoiling him a little, all this fussing probably does him little good and no harm. But it can—and often does—have an adverse effect on the owner and his attitude toward the dog. If he makes caring for the dog into an endless series of chores, he may in time become weary of the burdens he has saddled himself with. And resentful—resentful not only of the chores but of the dog himself. There is that danger. But whatever the faults of overconcern, they are infinitely better than the effects of neglect. If you are going to make a mistake with the old dog, let it be on the side of kindness. Nobody ever need be ashamed of pampering an old dog.

Owners almost always ask about the amount of exercise an old dog should or must have.

The obvious answer, it seems to me, is that the old dog should be allowed to decide for himself how much exercise he wants or needs. It is reasonable to encourage him to keep moving about and to offer him pleasant opportunities to limber up as he sees fit. But it is not a kindness to insist that he bestir himself when he would rather snooze, and it is certainly a mistake to imagine that forcing him to hike with you is somehow going to restore his fading muscles. If he enjoys walking with you, by all means take him whenever he wants to go. But be sensible about it. Turn back *before* he begins to tire so that he is not exhausted before he gets home. Many dogs are so glad to go for an outing and so anxious to please their owners that they will happily overdo the exercise. After they have rested a bit, their muscles will be so tight and sore that they will have difficulty in merely getting up and moving around the house. With some types of arthritis, even moderate exercise may have painful consequences, and since old Hector doesn't make the cause-effect connection, you may have to discourage him from taking walks that are going to make him uncomfortable the next day. If this problem seriously restricts his activity, your veterinarian will be able to provide some help to ease and minimize the discomfort.

Feeding—proper feeding—is a subject of such importance to the welfare of the dog throughout his life that I have thought it worthwhile to talk about it, emphatically and at length, elsewhere in this book. The principles, practices, and malpractices discussed there are all applicable here. And the benefits of sensible feeding continue to accrue. If you have had the foresight to regulate and control the dog's diet properly while he was young and if you do not have to contend with extraneous problems—obesity, for example—then feeding should not be a grave problem when the dog is old.

While they are active and healthy, dogs continue to thrive well on the diets they were accustomed to in their middle years. But when the dog is very old, dietary changes do sometimes become necessary either because of the weakening of the digestive system itself or because, in the treatment of a disease condition, certain food elements must be reduced or eliminated. In chronic kidney disease, for example, the amount of protein has to be sharply curtailed and so a nourishing low-protein or predigested protein diet is substituted for the usual one. Your veterinarian can devise a diet of this sort which you can prepare at home. Or, with less bother but at substantially higher cost, you can buy prescription diets which serve the same purpose. Switching the old dog from his familiar food to a strange one often requires large amounts of patience and persistence, but when his survival depends upon your success, you will manage it somehow.

Your veterinarian will be able to suggest a number of ways to make the transition as painless as possible for you and the dog.

If the old dog develops serious difficulties in his digestive system or if, in his dotage, the system simply fails to function adequately, it may be both kind and wise to return to the diet on which he was weaned. If the shift is made gradually, it can usually be accomplished without much resistance or disruption. Some types of digestive difficulties can be eliminated—or at least minimized—by putting the food through the old reliable household blender and thus reducing it to a consistency that makes it much more available to the digestive process. Food served this way may seem to you to be singularly unattractive, but to the dog's nose it is appealing. It is a convenient and effective way to provide a balanced diet and to avoid greater difficulties.

Fresh water should, of course, always be available to the dog. And as he grows older it becomes increasingly important to keep a record from time to time of the amount he drinks. During the heat of summer his fluid intake will naturally increase. But if there is a large or persistent variation from the normal amount, you should report it to your veterinarian. It might be a symptom of a developing problem which requires early treatment.

Vitamins and supplements are sometimes helpful and occasionally necessary. But less often than faddist, vitamin-popping owners think. Generally, so long as a dog is able to handle a sound, balanced diet, he will thrive without boosters. When the dog is on a restricted diet or when he has a disease condition that creates an imbalance of some sort, he may need some particular kind of supplement. But that is a matter for the veterinarian to decide. Not you. Dropping one of your pills in his dish now and then is neither right nor bright.

Housing the old dog isn't—or shouldn't be—a bothersome problem. Here again, it seems to me, the best practice is to make only the changes that are necessary to accommodate his infirmities, to make them as gradually as possible, and to avoid the fussy kind of *comforting* which may be intended to improve the quality of his life but more often turns out to be an unwelcome disruption of his familiar routine. He'd rather do it his way, and unless you know something that he doesn't, you shouldn't distress him by insisting that he change his style. You won't do thoughtless things to him. If he has always lived in an apartment where the temperature and humidity are closely controlled, you won't ship him off to Uncle Arthur while you spend Christmas week in Florida—if Uncle Arthur *knows* that it is good for the dog to sleep in his unheated garage. And you won't get sudden, whimsical notions. If he is a kennel dog, you won't decide one day that at his age he deserves the best, and install him in the old nursery with satin pillows.

When it does become necessary to change his living arrangements—as it will—you should do it as unobtrusively as possible. Little by little as he grows older, his bed should become softer and more resilient. He'll be spending more time there and, especially if he is a heavy dog, lying on a hard surface could cause callouses and sores at pressure points. If he becomes arthritic, you may be able to ease his discomfort by keeping his sleeping quarters a little warmer than they were in the past. And you may have to move his bed to a more convenient place so that he won't have to climb stairs every time he wants to snooze. Sometimes it is best to set up the new place as a *second* bed so that he can get used to it before the old one is removed.

Even with his reduced activity, he will usually be able to tolerate the normal variations in temperature that he has been accustomed to. But, as we have said, blizzards and the blistering noonday sun are not for old dogs. His thermostat doesn't respond as quickly as it did in his younger days, and he can be hurt by sudden or prolonged exposure to extreme temperatures. You'll have to discourage him from finding that out the hard way. Most dogs modify their ways to fit their strength and circumstances, but if you happen to have a determined old cuss who refuses to recognize his limitations, you may have to work a bit to teach him the virtues of moderation.

With the very old dog, hospitalization poses a problem to which there is simply no happy or satisfactory answer. All dogs are apprehensive in hospital surroundings and to some degree all are distressed by the strangeness of the place—the barking, the antiseptic smells, the cages, the white-coated attendants, the scent of strange animals. But old dogs, being less adaptable, are likely to have the most disturbing reactions. In extreme cases they may refuse to drink or sleep, and sometimes they may go on a complete hunger strike, pining for their owners and whining and barking inconsolably. When they are in such a state, treatment is always difficult and recovery is generally slowed.

For the owner the only workable, acceptable answer to the dilemma, it seems to me, is to try by all reasonable means to keep hospitalization to a minimum. Obviously, that doesn't mean that you can arbitrarily refuse to let the dog be hospitalized or that you will foolishly endanger the dog's life by resorting to half-measures at home. In many types of illness and injury you have no alternative: the dog *must* be hospitalized since there is no way that he can be properly treated elsewhere. But *if* there is a choice and *when* there is a choice, in my opinion it is always better to treat an old dog at home.

By that *if* and *when* I mean this: *If* the veterinarian is willing to let you take the dog home and care for him yourself, do it. He will point out the difficulties—medications that have to be measured and timed accurately; dressings that have to be changed; reports of reactions to be made; records to be kept. The veterinarian may expect a daily report at some outrageously early presurgery hour. Or you may have to take the dog back to the hospital every day for treatment. But if the veterinarian thinks that you *can* do the job and is willing to let you try, don't hesitate. Take the dog home with you. Whatever you lack in skill and dexterity will be more than compensated for by the benefits the dog will get from being in familiar surroundings.

And by *when* I mean simply that if the old dog *must* be hospitalized, you should take him home just as soon as the veterinarian is willing to release him in your care—for the same reasons. You may be nervous about assuming the responsibilities, you may have to learn to handle some messy jobs, and you may lose some sleep for a week or so. But you will have the satisfaction of knowing that the old boy is being given the best possible chance for a short, happy convalescence.

One thing above all you must provide for the very old dog: extra protection against the hazards and accidents to which he is exposed. Cautious as he may seem, by the time he gets into his dotage he has lost his old ability to fend for himself, and it becomes your responsibility to see that he doesn't get into predicaments from which he cannot extricate himself. Almost always he is at least partially blind and deaf, his responses are slow and uncertain, his strength and endurance have been greatly reduced. It is a mistake to assume that because he has become more staid and deliberate these last years he has also become wiser. On the contrary, he has become less capable, less alert, and less aware, weaker and more endangered than he has been since he was a puppy. He is, in fact, in his second puppyhood. And he is as vulnerable as he was then.

It is hard for most people to conceive of the difficulties that an old dog can stumble into. He can get into disastrous trouble in places where you would think it impossible for him to find trouble. Let me mention—just mention—a few of the scores of unbelievable incidents that I have seen in my own practice. The door from a bedroom to an upstairs terrace was left open. The old dog, wandering through the house, walked outside—where he had been hundreds of times—and injured himself fatally in a fall down a long flight of exterior stairs. He couldn't see the stairs. Or forgot they were there. Another, turned out in the back yard for his usual relief stroll one winter day, wandered out on thin, snow-covered ice on the pond and was lost. One old fellow, tied to the banisters of the porch where he was sunning, squeezed through a too-small opening, fell, and hanged himself in his own collar. And still another, a feeble old arthritic who could no longer patrol his yard, was left on a screened porch while his owner went to the village to shop. He was found there mangled when she returned. Apparently he had tried to bark off a large dog who had intruded in the yard; the invader had pushed open the latched door, and the proud old dog had been killed trying to defend the last bit of territory around his doorstep.

And always and forever there is the unending stream of old dogs who for years obediently stay on their owner's property—until one day they stray beyond the limits and are struck by an automobile. One case among hundreds: A fourteen-year-old brought to me a few months ago had been struck by a car a block from his home. And then, according to a witness, while he was crawling toward the safety of the curb, he was run over by a second car. Typically, the owner said, "Doctor, I can't understand it. He never leaves our yard. He was trained not to leave. He hasn't left the yard once in five years." What the owner failed to realize was that in five years an alert, well-trained animal had become a confused, befuddled old dog who was lost and frightened almost within sight of his own home. Incredibly, this stout old boy, broken and torn as he was, survived. But few dogs and few owners are so lucky.

Old dogs are wandering dogs. And if they venture a few yards beyond the patch of ground they still know, they are lost dogs. Frightened and disoriented, they turn first one way and then another, moving still further into a strange and terrifying world of vague shapes and booming sounds. And often, days and miles away, still searching for some familiar scent or sound that will lead them home, they die in accidents or of exposure and exhaustion. To me this seems the saddest and cruelest end of all—for the dog and for his owner.

The very old dog needs—must have—special care and protection. He deserves more than that. These are the years when he deserves all of the patience, the tolerance, the indulgence you can give him. He holds on with a kind of awkward tenacity. He is still anxious to please, but often slow to comprehend; willing to participate, but not always able to share the activities; reluctant to give up his old duties, but without the stamina to accomplish them. He means well. But he does what he will in his own wayward way. He is changeable and unpredictable—insistent, childish, perverse, angry, or amiable. He lives in a kind of half-world. He sees less, hears less, understands less. And heeds less. But if his world seems small and restricted to us, it is still sufficient for him. He accepts it as it is. And seems happy with it.

He is a trial and a comfort. Sometimes an exasperating comfort. And if, when patience wears thin, you must scold the old boy, you scold him gently and with no real hope of repentance or improvement. For you know and he knows that you really don't mean what you say. You both know that you will forgive his failures, excuse his lapses, tolerate his nuisances.

What else could you do?

A woman I know well has a four-pound toy Manchester, named Perry Mason for some forgotten reason. She lives near me, and ever since her husband gave her the dog eighteen years ago, I've been consulting, on-hand veterinarian. From the beginning Perry was, within the limitations of his size, an obstreperous and strident guardian of the house. Too endlessly strident, in fact. Years ago, with the connivance and urging of the husband, I debarked the dog, telling his mistress a black half-truth—that the dog had lost his voice. It was a very minor operation which reduced his piercing yelps to a series of vigorous but nearly soundless exhalations of air. But the woman discovered our duplicity (her husband told her, I think) and was furious—until she was convinced that the silent explosions were as satisfying to Perry as the old ear-splitters. He remained lord of the manse, and even now, when he is deaf and half-blind, he manages to strut with minor, arthritic dignity.

But the woman's husband died last year, and without his restraining presence, Perry has been pampered rotten. Not surprisingly, he has been permitted to abandon his comfortable basket and to sleep on the foot of his mistress's bed. Because of his size and the infirmities of age, he has to be lifted onto the bed when he retires and handed down when he gets up. Worse, his kidneys are not what they once were. Recently the woman admitted to me that it had become a regular two o'clock ritual for Perry to dance on her until she got up, took him to the kitchen for watering, and brought him back to bed. That, I thought, was an imposition. It was a simple abuse of the woman's kindness and consideration. And though I have the greatest love and respect for the woman, I exploded. I was firm with her. I was vehement.

"That's nonsense! That's simply ridiculous! Put the damn dog back in his basket, Mother!"

"Oh, George. . . . Be quiet," she said. "It pleases him . . . and me, too."

And I think she's right. Again.

V
A Prudent Program for Maintenance

Veterinarians can be almost as vain as people and as proud of their good works as others are of theirs. All of us in the profession collect and treasure memories of heroic operations, nick-of-time insights, desperate efforts that succeeded. But more and more I find that what remains with me and nourishes my ego best is not the recollection of occasional gratifying successes in emergencies but the thought that I have been able to convince a good many clients of the wisdom and value of timely preventive care and treatment for their animals. That doesn't sound like much to be proud of. But as the old lady said of the hummingbird, it's good—what there is of it.

Like health services for humans, veterinary medicine has, I think, been too closely geared to handling problems at the emergency stage. Our concern has been too exclusively centered on perfecting ways to cope with life-threatening situations after they arise, and far too little effort has gone into developing and promoting programs designed to maintain good health. On neither level has progress been as soon and steady as it should have been, but preventive care is still lagging, still being shamefully neglected. Today, in my opinion, the development of planned, practical programs in this area is one of the most urgently necessary steps in the advance of veterinary medicine.

It isn't going to be easy to change old attitudes and established habits. Everybody—nearly everybody—knows that the veterinarian's function is to treat sick animals. Most people consult him for that purpose. And for no other. If you ask, a dog owner will tell you, of course, that the veterinarian could and would perform a far more useful and humane service by keeping the animal well rather than by preventing him from dying. And in the abstract they *believe* that, too. But still they wait until the dog is sick before they take him to the veterinarian. That's the custom. That's the way it has always been. And no matter what he says he thinks, it is a rare owner who consults his veterinarian while his dog is well.

The blame doesn't rest entirely on the owners, either. The veterinarians themselves have not been notably active in promoting and encouraging maintenance programs. There have been a few lonely pioneers in the field. William Whittick, D.V.M., of Toronto, has worked indefatigably to devise a sound regimen for old dogs and to get others to develop similar programs. But most practitioners have been slow to follow his lead. And with reasons. A veterinarian is often hesitant to suggest a plan which a wary client could misconstrue as a scheme to bind him to some sort of annual fee arrangement. Everything is already predated, automatically billed, and outrageously expensive—and *now,* health insurance for the dog? For the veterinarian there is also the problem of time. He is busy, and working up an individual program of this sort commonly takes a considerable amount of time—for which the veterinarian is poorly paid simply because he finds it difficult to charge fees on a realistic time-cost basis. Even though he would like to do more of this kind of work, he feels that he can't afford it. And typically, when the opportunity to discuss such a program does turn up, it is often at precisely the moment when the waiting room is bulging with sick and injured animals in need of immediate attention.

In the hectic routine of emergency treatment in the veterinarian's day, there is too little opportunity to practice medicine for maintenance. But chances do appear—unexpectedly, unpredictably and (I hope and believe this is more than wishful thinking) more frequently than they did a few years ago. And I have found that a fairly agile and determined veterinarian can sometimes turn these chance encounters into good medicine.

Unpredictably, I say. And unabashedly I give you an example from my own practice.

One unusually busy morning several years ago there appeared in the examining room a patient entirely unknown to me—a six- or seven-year-old Airedale with a wart on his nose. He was accompanied by an owner (and I tell you this reluctantly, knowing that you will think it a preposterous lie) who also had a wart on his nose. He also had a smile-making name, but I'll spare you that. Call him Mr. Johns.

The dog's wart was no problem, but after it had been decided that it had to be removed, it became apparent that Mr. Johns had more than warts on his mind. He sidled around to his question rather awkwardly. "I was thinking, Doctor . . . I was thinking that Rex [that figured] . . . Rex is in pretty good shape, I guess. But it seems to me he's beginning to show his age. Slowing down a little. I was wondering if there was some kind of program for a dog like him. Like the one my doctor gave to me. Maybe you have one already written out I could take? You see, I like to keep old Rex in good shape and . . ."

The tempo was slow, but it was the kind of music I like. And for a veterinarian prone to lecture his clients on the value of a maintenance program, it was not a request to be ignored. Rex's wart was no urgent matter, so we arranged an appointment for him to have it removed at the end of office hours a few days later. The operation was totally uneventful (a local anesthetic and a single suture) and unimportant. But it did give us the time and opportunity to work out a maintenance program for Rex. And that *was* important.

There is, of course, no convenient *Universal Maintenance Program* neatly printed and stashed away in a drawer of your veterinarian's desk. Just as there is no sheet your doctor can hand you to solve your particular problems and enhance your hopes for a long and comfortable life. But I can assure you that a worthwhile program *can* be worked out for your dog—the canine equivalent of the Prudent Program which I hope and assume your doctor has prepared for you.

I'd like to tell you a little more about Rex. Not because the story is in any way remarkable, but because it is *not* remarkable. And not because your veterinarian is going to set up the same program for your dog. He won't. But he is likely to approach the problem in a similar fashion. And the result is more than likely to be the same—the development of a sensible, practical maintenance program that, barring major catastrophe, will see your dog through to a reasonably active, healthy, pain-free old age.

So here is Rex. I don't have a history for him yet. Mr. Johns has just moved to my parish and of course he didn't think of bringing Rex's medical record with him. But he appears to be a sensible old gentleman. As a matter of fact, since he actually came in to suggest the program, he already stands well up on my list. He recalls that Rex did have some shots, but he is not sure what kind or when or how many, and he certainly hasn't had any in years. But then, he hasn't been sick, either, so there wasn't any reason to take him to the veterinarian. (You weren't expecting a perfect client, were you?) Rex is six years old. Mr. Johns is pretty sure of that. He couldn't be seven yet. And he is a little overweight. He has been gaining a little in the last couple of years. And, oh yes, occasionally he holds his head to one side. Mr. Johns wants to know if that means there might be something wrong. There are a lot more questions I have to ask—you've been through a sampling of them a few pages back—and Mr. Johns fields them well. When we are through, Rex has a fuller and more reliable history than most newcomers.

With that in hand we were ready to consider what else was needed—the physical examination, the tests, the basic information necessary to work up a program for the present and to establish base-line data for the future. And we talked about the cost. Mr. Johns was not in the money-is-of-no-consequence class. So we considered what must be done immediately, what was important for the record, what could be done later as occasion arose. Since Rex was obviously in sound condition generally, we chose to take a conservative, middle course. I'll tell you about the plan we worked out. And what it cost.

It is always risky to talk about fees, and any veterinarian who does should be careful to remind the reader that the figures he gives are based solely on his own arithmetic in his own locality at a particular time. Every veterinarian works in his own microeconomy, and his charges are necessarily based on the costs and prices he has to live with. So fees vary, as they must. Those suggested here are not drawn from holy writ. But in my particular here-and-now they seem to me to be sensible, fair charges for the work performed. I use specific figures here because I think cost is a factor that most people have to consider and because I find it awkward and evasive to talk about these procedures without indicating what the cost is likely to be. Even if my clients don't ask, I tell them. I see no reason to be more reticent with you.

This is the way it worked out for Rex. The procedures would be essentially the same for any dog without special problems.

First there is the general physical examination. It includes taking a complete history, which has already been mentioned. In addition, every area of the dog's body is examined methodically and carefully, with specialized instruments where necessary: the eyes, the nose, the teeth and gums, the mouth and throat, the other natural openings of the body. The dog's coat and skin are thoroughly examined from tip to tail. The feet and nails are carefully examined. If there are any lumps, cysts, warts, or other growths, their nature, location, and size are noted. The charge for this examination is $10.

A urinalysis is performed, primarily to determine the efficiency of the kidney function. It may also reflect problems in other organs such as the liver. Charge: $6.

A blood test is needed. The number, type, and condition of the blood cells often reflect problems long before overt symptoms are observed. And so a red and white blood count is made. Another test is used to determine hemoglobin levels and the proportion of cells to serum in the circulating blood. In addition, the blood is tested for certain elements which reflect the function of the liver and kidneys. These tests require specialized, expensive equipment, and they are often time-consuming. The charge for the battery of blood tests is the largest single item: About $30.

A fecal examination is made to determine whether internal parasites are present. Charge: $3.

And, since the dog must be kept at the veterinarian's place for the day—and sometimes overnight—for the examination and series of tests, there will be a hospitalization charge. In our case: $8.

If the examination by stethoscope suggests that it is advisable to perform an EKG to determine the quality of the dog's heartbeat, that will be done. Even if there is no irregularity, I urge that it be taken since it is extremely useful to have a tracing of the normal heartbeat to compare with later EKGs should an abnormal condition develop. It costs $10.

And if during the examination it has been necessary to take x-rays, that would be an additional $15.

So, by this reckoning, the total comes to $82—or, without the x-rays—to $67. That's not a magnificent sum. Nor an insignificant one, either. In this case, as it happened, Rex turned out to be in splendidly normal condition. The only thing I found which needed attention was a minor ear irritation for which I supplied a remedy. But we did have assurance that there were no hidden conditions developing into major problems, and I did have a detailed record which was to serve as a useful reference many times thereafter. Those two things alone, I think, are worth more than the cost. But in cases where we do find latent problems, an examination of this sort always saves valuable time and prevents needless suffering. Not infrequently, it also saves the dog's life.

The following week, when the results of the tests were all in, Mr. Johns and I had another session to review them and to plan the program he had originally asked about. In the past I have sometimes prepared a report for the owner, a summary of the results of the examination and a list of suggestions for the care of the dog in the future. But I have come to doubt the usefulness of such a document. Often, it seems to me, it encourages an attitude of passive acceptance on the part of the owner. He accepts it routinely, folds it carefully, and when he gets home, I have a feeling, files it away with the receipts for the license fees. I'd rather spend more time with the owner, discuss the dog's condition with him, answer his questions, and make specific suggestions on the basis of the owner's own needs and experience. I have a pad and pencil for him, and what he writes he will read and remember. Mr. Johns was a knowledgeable man, but he took away a handful of notes and reminders.

1) *Annual checkup.* We agreed (or agreed again) that sick or well Rex would be brought in for a checkup

once a year. And he has been. Once we removed an accumulation of tartar that had started a gum infection. Another time we discovered a small anal tumor, possibly malignant, and took it out. Later there was an infection of the prostate which we were able to clear up before it became serious.

2) *Regular observation.* We talked a bit about the importance of keeping an eye on the dog's general appearance and his daily activities, of being aware of changes and of reporting any that were abrupt or unusual. With Mr. Johns this was no problem, of course. But with some people it is. It takes a Dutch-uncle lecture to convince them of the importance of seeing.

3) *Home examination.* A careful hand inspection at least once a month is simple, sensible insurance. What that means is discussed elsewhere in this book. With Rex on the table, Mr. Johns and I went through the whole exercise, from tooth and tongue to tail and toe. You'd be wise to have your veterinarian give you a demonstration too.

4) *Food.* Nothing is more important in a maintenance program than the proper control of diet. As you will see in the section on food. Rex, as it happened, was gaining weight by being allowed as much dehydrated meal as he wanted. We reduced the amount by 25 percent until he dropped back to his normal weight three or four months later, and then increased it slightly to a maintenance level. Since then it has been reduced still further to keep him in trim. In time he was eating about half as much as he did when he was a young dog.

5) . . . *and drink.* It's important to monitor the fluid intake too. Mr. Johns hadn't been doing that. Few people do. A persistent need for more than the usual amount of fluid may indicate the presence of diabetes, kidney disease, and other problems. Any change should be reported to the veterinarian. Promptly.

6) *Exercise.* An area of much concern and much dis-

pute for which there is no fits-all-sizes formula answer. You'll find it discussed elsewhere in this book. Rex had once had the run of a yard, but in his new unfenced location he had been restricted to leash walking except for weekend jaunts and outings. The change seemed to bother him, so Mr. Johns agreed to rig up a glider-on-a-line arrangement, which improved matters. Later he fenced in a run for Rex, and that was still better.

7) *Environment.* As the dog grows older, the prudent rule-of-thumb program is to reduce his exposure to extremes. Like most Airedales, Rex was contemptuous of weather conditions. In winter he was happy to go to sleep on a snowdrift and in summer he would run endlessly in the noontime sun. At first it was enough to discourage him from indulging in excesses. Later his frolics had to be more rigidly forbidden.

8) *Physical protection.* Owners commonly make the disastrous mistake of thinking that as a dog grows older he becomes wise and wary, less endangered by accidents and street hazards. The opposite is true, and the reasons for that are discussed at length in other sections of this book. Rex's outside activities were controlled and supervised. He was not permitted to roam the neighborhood.

9) *Grooming.* As a dog grows older, health and comfort become more important than style and fashion. Rex was kept well plucked and barbered as he had always been. A long coat protects a dog against the cold, but it is nonsense to say that it also insulates him against the heat. Dogs are obviously more comfortable with a summer cut, and when it grows in again, the new coat is normally healthy and lustrous. Bathing is often the only way to get rid of city grime, but dogs who live in better circumstances do well with regular combing and brushing and only an occasional bath. Dogs are commonly washed more often than they want to be, need to be, or should be. Good foot care, which is often neglected, is more important. Nails that are allowed to grow too long make walking

painful, often cut toes and create infections and even cause painful abrasions when the dog intends only to scratch for the pleasure of it.

10) *Change and routine.* Dogs live patterned lives. They habituate themselves to their circumstances, and once they have established a routine, they thrive on it. And the older they get the less they welcome change. Abrupt changes in his routine make an old dog uneasy and uncomfortable, and when modifications are necessary, he should be eased into the transition as gently as possibly and not thrust into it suddenly.

11) *Travel.* Whatever his custom has been. If he rides well, take him with you as long as he is able to get around reasonably well. But you will, of course, have to make more frequent rest stops. And you'll have to watch him carefully when he is out of the car.

12) *If you can't take him with you.* Leaving him becomes difficult. Make the best arrangements you can. But go. If he has been accustomed to staying with a neighbor or at your sister's house, that will probably continue to work well—at least until he becomes crotchety. If you must get a sitter, try to get a conscientious and dependable friend. A friend of *his.* Have the sitter spend as much time as he can with him. Be sure that the dog has everything that he needs and that all the old familiars and comfortables are there for him. And give him a long, large greeting when you get back, especially if he seems put out with you.

This, in outline, is a *Prudent Plan*—the essential elements of a program designed to maintain health and to minimize the premature and preventable problems of aging. This program was intended for Rex, and for him it was sufficient. With the variations necessary to fit particular needs and circumstances, a similar regimen can be worked out for any dog. Such a plan is ordinarily so simple that it is almost an overstatement to call it a program. There is nothing about it that a responsible owner should find difficult, demanding or even time-consuming. And yet I am convinced that a precautionary program no more elaborate than the one proposed here will often add comfortable years to a dog's life. I am equally sure that the owner who has enough concern and foresight to sit down with his veterinarian and work out such a program will not only be doing his dog a great service. In the long run he will also be saving himself worry, regret—and money.

And Rex—what about old Rex? At fourteen, he's in fine shape. He's both a good example and a poor one. If I were making him up just to illustrate the value of a maintenance program, I think I would have added a touch of drama toward the end. It would have been persuasive to report that during one of his routine annual examinations we discovered an unsuspected and potentially fatal condition which we were able to treat and cure just in time. But so far nothing of that sort has happened. It seems a bit dull to have to say that the notations for his last checkup read a flat normal, normal, normal. Mr. Johns does complain, however, that the old boy is becoming unbearably dignified. Having Rex in the house, he says, is like having a bishop on permanent loan.

VI When Hector Is Sick

There is nothing like a sick dog to shake an owner's confidence in his ability to cope. Kin Hubbard, the cracker-barrel philosopher, once said, "No one feels as helpless as the owner of a sick goldfish." I suppose he was right. But in my practice, at least, fish keepers seem to accept their problems stoically. Dog owners don't. They worry. They worry a lot about what they can do, what they should do, what they shouldn't do. They may not feel as totally helpless as Hubbard's goldfish fellow, but they almost always need more help and reassurance.

Dogs being as durable and sick-proof as they generally are, many an owner of a middle-aged dog has never even had to give him a pill. When a sturdy, problem-free family fixture unaccountably becomes a sick old dog, the owner suddenly discovers that he doesn't know a thing about how to take care of him. And the person who never had a question to ask the veterinarian immediately has a rash of urgent inquiries that have to be answered on the spot. "How will I know when . . .", "What will I do if . . .", "When will he be . . .", "What does it mean if . . .", "Won't it be hard to . . ." And at the end there is almost always the sad plaint, "Oh, if he could only *tell* us where it hurts." Yes, indeed. If only he could. If only Dr. Dolittle were here.

A sick dog is not a catastrophe. He is a problem. The fact that you don't know what is wrong with him or what to do about it—and you won't—doesn't mean that you are facing a calamity. There is no need to go into a tizzy about it. Whatever it is, the chances are good that something can be done about it and that it won't end in disaster. And whatever it is, the chances also are that it won't go away if you ignore it. The sensible thing to do is to find out what it is and what can be done about it. And the sensible way to do that is to get in touch with your veterinarian. Not your neighbor. Not your father-in-law. Your veterinarian.

How quickly you must talk to your veterinarian depends, of course, on what is happening to the dog. Some conditions are obviously so acute that there can be no question about them. There are also less obvious emergency situations—you'll find them in the discussion of panic-button problems—when you would be remiss if you didn't call your veterinarian at three o'clock in the morning. Others will wait until the office opens in the morning. And there are even a few that can be held over until your day off on Thursday. But the rule is: If you are in doubt, sooner is better.

Take a for-instance: Hector doesn't eat his usual evening meal. He sniffs and mopes off to his corner for the rest of the night. That's unusual, but no cause for alarm. But when you get up the next morning, you see that Hector has vomited a time or two and doesn't seem to be interested in you or in anything else. He is a sick dog and looks it, but— While you clean up the mess, you think about what you should do. It's an urgent day at the office —it always is—so you decide to get dressed and have your coffee and see how things are then. So he doesn't seem any *worse* and you go to the office and your wife calls and says he is vomiting again and is trembling badly and you don't know what to do really but you'll come home early and we'll see then but by that time the veterinarian must have left his office and you'll call him first thing in the morning.

That's the way to do everything wrong. By the next morning (as it turned out in the actual case I am reporting here) you have a dog in a critical diabetic depression, and it is touch and go whether the veterinarian can save him. If you had *called* the veterinarian the first morning, he would have told you to bring the dog in immediately. The veterinarian would have been able to give the dog an injection to stabilize his condition while tests were being made and you could have been in and out of his office in fifteen minutes. You might have been as much as an hour late getting to the office, but by that evening you would have known that you had a live dog under treatment instead of discovering the next day that you had a half-dead dog who might or might not survive. A day can make that much difference.

The moral of this is short, simple, and obvious: Call your veterinarian. If the dog is sick enough to make you wonder if you should wait and see, he is *too* sick for you to wait and see. Call. Dogs die of a great variety of conditions that cannot be cured or controlled. But one of the major causes of death is entirely preventable. It is delay.

Your first and most important duty, then, is to see that the dog's condition is promptly and properly diagnosed. That is a job for your veterinarian, I repeat, and not for you. It may be that you have had half a dozen dogs and that you have had much more than the usual amount of experience in caring for them. And there is no doubt that you have what is called good common sense. But it takes more than the best common sense to make a diagnosis; it requires specialized training, skill, experience, knowledge, and facilities which you simply don't have. You can guess. Anybody can. But in the kind of guessing game you will be playing the odds are always that you won't win. And the dog can only lose.

Common sense is an uncommonly popular gift and much has been said and written in praise of it. And properly so. It is often the best—and sometimes the only—alternative we have for knowledge. In its place it is useful and necessary. But misused or overused—as it often is—it can be lethally dangerous. Everybody you know is certain that he himself has sound common sense—and he can instantly name a dozen people who haven't. It sometimes seems to me that half the mistakes I hear about in my office are prefaced with the absolving phrase, "Well, it just seemed like common sense to—" And perhaps it did, but far too often it turned out to be something quite different. It is always dangerous to try to use a substitute when only skill will serve. Common sense is of no use whatsoever to a person who is getting on a bicycle for the first time. And it is not a tool you can safely use to diagnose your dog's condition.

There is at least one good thing to be said about caring for a sick dog: It is generally much less difficult than you expect it to be. It does require care and diligence and attention. And you will be expected to follow instructions exactly, observe what is happening accurately, and report what you see reliably. But you won't be required to have either the skills of a registered nurse or the wisdom of Solomon. Or even that of a veterinarian. However sick your dog may be, there are only a limited number of things you can be asked to do for him. You will be *told* what you are to do, and you will be *shown* how you are to do it. If you are asked to do more than a very few simple things, you will be given written instructions. Even after you get the dog home, you are not alone with him and his problems. You have a telephone and a veterinarian at the other end of it.

It is a strange thing (I think) but I often discover that an owner thinks that to take care of one sick little dog properly he should be qualified to handle all of the ills of dogdom. That's really not necessary. All he needs to know is how to take care of a few small problems of one small dog at one particular time. There was once a man (or at least there was a fable about a man) who kept right on gathering and eating mushrooms even though many people were being poisoned by those they picked in the woods. His neighbors said to the man, "You are a fool. There are a thousand species of mushrooms out there. Many of them are poisonous—and you can't *possibly* know a thousand mushrooms." "No, I don't," said the man, gathering still more. "I know only six—and every one of them is delicious." Moral: You don't have to know everything. And you can easily learn the half-dozen things you *do* need to know to take care of your dog.

How you rate your ability to cope often has a direct bearing on how and where your dog will be treated and on how well and how quickly he recovers. When he is critically ill or has been seriously injured, he will have to be kept, for a time at least, in the hospital. But with less acute illnesses, you and your veterinarian will have to decide whether the dog is to remain in the hospital or can be cared for at home. Hospitalization is a trauma for most dogs—and particularly for an old dog—and a clinical atmosphere is never as conducive to quick recovery as familiar home surroundings. But if you have an exaggerated idea of what is expected of you, if you are afraid that you won't be able to take care of the dog properly, if you think that you are likely to make a terrible blunder that will jeopardize the dog's very life, you will certainly choose to leave him in the hospital. And that, I think, is usually a mistake. It is true, of course, that there are owners who are so nervous, so uncertain, and so uncommonly inept that no veterinarian would risk leaving a sick dog in their care. But they are few. If your veterinarian thinks that you *can* take care of your dog, believe him. In my opinion an old dog should never be kept in the hospital unless there is some clear and pressing reason why he cannot be treated at home.

In actual practice it often happens that the procedures that at first seem to the owner most disturbing or frightening are easily learned and soon accepted as part of the routine. To go back for a moment to the case of the diabetic dog: After he had been in the hospital for a week, his condition was sufficiently stabilized for him to be taken home. He was not *cured,* of course, but he was ready to begin living the near-normal life that all diabetics must accept. But the continuing daily care which he needed posed problems for his owners. His exercise had to be regulated, his urine tested regularly for sugar, his diet rigidly controlled (which meant that he could never be allowed off the leash outdoors)—and he had to have a daily injection of insulin.

The owners' response was an immediate, emphatic, horrified *No.* All the business about the diet, the exercise, the tests—all that the owners were willing to undertake. But *not* the injections. "I couldn't. I simply couldn't. Not even once. And every day? Never!" But when they understood that their only choice was between learning to give the dog insulin shots or leaving him for euthanasia, they went home to ponder overnight. When they came in the next day, they said simply, "We're here to bite the bullet."

For the remaining days the dog was in the hospital, one or the other of the owners came in to practice giving the shot. They winced, but they learned quickly, and after they took the dog home, he continued to do well. And so did the needle pushers. When other owners were tempted to destroy good dogs, I used to send them to consult with my experts. Over the years they saved the lives of many dogs.

People rise to cope with difficult problems. It is often the simple little procedures that baffle and frustrate the owner. Many kinds of medicine, for example, are given in liquid form. Getting a distasteful liquid into a reluctant dog is no problem at all for your veterinarian. But it is for you. If you fail to remind the good doctor that old Hector has never been sick for a day in his life, he may assume that you know how to give the stuff to the dog—and thus innocently involve you in a protracted test of mind and muscle with Hector. If you ask your veterinarian, he'll tell you several ways to save face and avoid spilled medicine.

If the medicine is, by good fortune, bland or odorless enough to be inoffensive to the dog, you may be able to palm it off on him in his food. Try a little *with* a little—to minimize the loss if he refuses to cooperate. Ice cream is a powerful temptation, and Hector may surprise you by lapping up a sundae made with a concoction that seems absolutely revolting to you.

And when ruses fail—as they often do—there is always the standard this-hurts-me-more-than-it-does-you method. Measure the medicine into a small paper cup and put it where it will be within reach at the critical time. Position old Hector in a corner or against the wall where he can't back away from you. Stand in front of him—or sit, if he is a small dog or insists on lying down to take his medicine. Tilt his head back and with your left hand make a pouch by pulling his lips away from his teeth on the side next to you. Pour in the medicine from the cup which—if you have planned well—is conveniently at your right. But not more than a swallow—a tablespoonful—at a time. Keep his head back, stroke his throat, hold his mouth shut—and down it goes. Usually. Do it all as smoothly and firmly as you can. Reruns get harder. Fortunately, this is easier than it reads—like tying a shoelace. If it sounds like a contortionist's routine, you might try it on Hector while he is in good health. It is not likely that he will approve of this strange new embrace, but it'll do him no harm, and the practice may someday stand you in good stead. But seeing is always best. When your veterinarian hands you the prescription, ask him to demonstrate the trick.

Pills and capsules offer the opportunity for a great range of deceitful practices. They can be hidden in a little chopped meat. Or inserted in a piece of frankfurter. Or wrapped in cheese. Or served as a fancy liver paté on cracker. One ingenious client of mine folds the capsules in little chicken-skin envelopes and freezes the whole course of treatment. Her dog begs for them like Sunday treats.

And all pills go well with candy, of course. Sweets now and then can't hurt a healthy dog, and for the pill giver, candy is hard to beat. The soft-center chocolate was invented for your purpose. A marshmallow will conceal the bitterest dose. And if you drop a broken bit of hard candy on the floor for Hector, and then another, and then a pill, and then another piece of candy, Hector will often vacuum them all up and wait for more.

But after about the third day, or after he has had the luck to unwrap one of these bitter little gifts, Hector may begin to suspect this spate of unusual generosity. He will check the offering carefully, and if his nose tells him that it is loaded, he will either refuse it altogether or take the time to peel off the good part and leave the pill. You will have to polish your act by adding prestidigitation to simple deceit. With elaborate ostentation prepare three delightful treats—cheese balls on crackers today, let's say—with the pill artfully concealed in Number Two. Show him that you have lots of goodies, and when you have his undivided attention, offer him the first for his approval. He will inspect it carefully and be surprised and delighted to find that it is innocent. Show him that there are still two more to come. One in each hand. If you manage it properly, he'll bolt down Number Two to get to the third before you change your mind.

But some dogs—and you may be one of the chosen owners—flatly refuse to play the pill-in-a-paté game. When guile fails, you'll have to use a more direct method. Put the dog in a corner where he can't back away from you. Grasp his muzzle with your left hand, tilt his head back, and with your thumb on one side and fingers on the other squeeze his lips against his teeth until he opens his mouth. You won't have to apply much pressure. Holding the pill between thumb and forefinger of your right hand, use the bottom of the hand to push down his lower jaw and open his mouth wide. Drop the pill on the back of his tongue and with your finger or thumb push it as far back into his throat as you can. Release your grip enough to let him close his mouth, but keep his head up. He has to swallow, and if you have put the pill far enough back in his mouth, it will go down.

There are dozens of innovative ways to give a dog a pill. But not all of them are practical. One Saturday night, years ago, my uncle called to ask how to get a pill into his dog. Late that afternoon, he explained, he had taken his dog to the veterinarian who had prescribed some pills. But it wasn't until medication time that evening that my uncle realized that he had neglected to ask the veterinarian how he was to persuade the dog to swallow the pill. He called the veterinarian at his home and, judging by the background sounds, interrupted a lively party. When my uncle asked how to handle his problem, there was a noticeable pause and then a booming voice. "Whitney—you have a chandelier, haven't you? Well, Whitney, the thing for you to do is to climb up on the chandelier and get it swinging. That will attract the dog's attention. You wait there until he runs underneath and barks up at you. Then it's easy. You just drop the pill right down his throat." And the veterinarian hung up. My uncle has a great sense of humor, too, and he gets along fine with his new veterinarian.

Veterinarians are busy. They have other small faults, too. One of them is a tendency to think that the client understands what they are talking about as long as he keeps nodding his head and saying "Yep . . . Yep . . . Yep." It is sometimes difficult to know whether an amiable client is absorbing what he is being told or is merely being agreeable. You won't be helping the doctor a bit by hearing him out to the end before you tell him that he lost you away back at the beginning. If you don't clearly understand what the veterinarian means, tell him so. Right then. There is always another, plainer way he can say what he has in mind. If you don't know how to do what you are expected to do, ask him. He will tell you. Even better, he may be able to *show* you. If the instructions seem complicated, write them down or have him write them out, and get them straight. And when you get home and find that you can't read your writing (or his), don't guess whether it was twice a day or every two days that you were to give the dog that pill. Call.

Strange things happen. I once explained to a client that her dog would have to be given pills for quite a time—two in the morning and two in the afternoon. And, knowing that the woman tended to be vague and forgetful, I scribbled a reminder for her: "Two—AM, Two—PM." I didn't hear from her for a week or so, and when she called she said the dog was doing fine. But if it was all right with me, she would like to make a change. It was easy to give the dog his pills in the afternoon, she said, but getting up to give him more pills at 2 A.M. was killing her.

Someday when you call your veterinarian, he is going to ask if your dog has been running a fever. You shouldn't sound as though you were surprised that a dog has such a thing as temperature or that you might be expected to know what it is.

You *can* take a dog's temperature at home. You should have a rectal thermometer in the house, and that is the one to use. Shake it down until you are sure that the reading is below 100° F. Put a little Vaseline on it and with a gentle twirling motion insert it until the bulb is at least an inch inside the dog's anus. Most thermometers register quickly, but to be on the safe side leave it in place for three minutes. Wipe it clean with a tissue and read it.

Don't worry about the 98.6° mark. That's for people. Normal temperature for most dogs is near 101° F., but your dog's everyday temperature may vary a bit from this statistical average. And the time of day you take it may make a slight difference too. Like yours, his temperature is likely to be a little below normal in the morning and a little above it later in the day.

When you take a sick dog to the veterinarian's office, the good doctor will have to supplement what he sees with background information from you. He'll ask questions. It will help him if you are prepared to answer them clearly and accurately and it will save everybody's time if you can do that without stopping to rummage around in the scattered recollections of the last few days.

Certainly the veterinarian will want to know *when* the dog got sick. And by that he means when you noticed that something was wrong. Most people are tempted to fudge this question a little because they are ashamed to confess that the dog may have been sick three or four days before he was brought in. It will help if you tell the truth, even if you lose a little face. And unless the dog was obviously and acutely ill, it is no great discredit to you if you hoped for a day or so that he really didn't have a doctor-size problem. After all, you yourself don't rush to your physician the first day you feel under the weather.

The veterinarian will almost certainly ask about the dog's appetite. What and how much and how well has the dog been eating? Has he been taking the usual amount of fluids? How much? And by fluids he means all liquids, of course, not just water.

He'll also ask if the dog has been having regular bowel movements and urinating normally. And if there has been any change in the color or consistency of the stools. The usual answer to these questions is a shrug and a vague well-he's-been-going-out-and-I-guess . . . But if your dog has been sick, you *should* know about these functions.

Has the dog been nauseated? Has he vomited? How often? How violently? Was there anything unusual about the appearance of the vomit? Has he been unsteady on his feet? Had problems going up or down stairs?

And the veterinarian is very likely to ask you to try to think of any unusual event or circumstance that might possibly have a bearing on the problem. Has the dog been loose or away from home recently? Has he been where he might get garbage or carrion or stale food? Has he had access to a place where something is being cleaned or scrubbed down? Where there is antifreeze solution? Paint or paint chips? Could he have come in contact with a sick dog someplace? Have you seen one around the neighborhood recently?

Questions of this sort are important and you should spend time thinking about them and others like them before you plump old Hector down on the examining table. What you don't think of mentioning may be the clue that the veterinarian needs.

When you take over as resident nurse and medical officer, your bedside manner becomes important. If you let old Hector discover that you are tense and apprehensive, he is likely to respond promptly by becoming uneasy and suspicious. He will be a much more cooperative patient if you go about the routine of caring for him calmly and cheerfully. He wants to please, and you can often *persuade* him to help you through the unpleasant part of the business. But threats and force almost always lead to a balking refusal or a wrestling match. Don't try to sneak up on him and get the job done before he knows what's happening. He knows, and it won't work. Go about what has to be done confidently and gently, and with as much dispatch as you can manage. But don't rush ahead and botch the job if you can wait a minute and then do it properly. Give him a little rest and a lot of reassurance as often as you can. Don't fight with him when you can reason with him. Speak softly—and carry a small stick of candy.

Your veterinarian will take all the time necessary to explain your dog's problem and to give you specific, detailed instructions about the care he needs. But he hasn't the time to give you a beginner's course in the methods of home dog care. He will omit what he assumes you know, and he won't try your patience by dwelling on the obvious. He'd be a tedious old bore if he did, the Polonius of the veterinary profession.

This Polonius, however, will risk a few more brief precepts:

Don't guess about anything. Ask.

Don't fuss. Make the dog as comfortable as you can, but don't hover over him. Too much attention will disturb him more than it comforts him.

Follow instructions. Two pills every eight hours is not one pill every four hours.

Don't *adjust* the medication. Don't increase, decrease, or discontinue the medicine because it *seems* that . . . If something does seem to be wrong, tell the veterinarian.

Don't let your neighbor persuade you to give Hector a little bit of the medicine that was so good for *her* dog.

Keep a written record. When you talk to the veterinarian, he'll ask when, how much, how long, how often.

Report all unusual or unexpected happenings immediately. Don't wait to see if they are *serious* or if they happen again.

Keep him clean. Keep his place clean. Have disposable cloths on hand. Change bandages or dressings as instructed, not when you think they need to be changed. Wash soiled areas promptly. Discard soiled cloths immediately or wash them in chlorine antiseptic.

Don't think that everything is back to normal the

first time the dog scratches at the door and asks to go out.

Don't pity yourself. Other people have had sicker dogs. And cared for them longer.

Avoid *common sense.* Use good judgment instead.

VII
Veterinarians . . . and Their Clients

Nearly half a century ago there lived in Hollywood a stock character called Ole Vet. You can still catch a glimpse of him between the antiperspirants on almost any channel that's on the air between 1:30 and 5:30 A.M. He's unmistakable in his way, but you'll have to watch for him.

Ole Vet was played by any one of a number of character actors, all of whom had mastered a single role—the gimpy, unshaven, lovably alcoholic, plastic-faced vet who opens his mouth wide to think, squints through steel-rims, scratches his cheek stubble with his thumb and begins all lines, of whatever import, with a drawled South-in-the-mouth "Wa-a-a-al . . ." There was only one costume and all the players, great or small, wore it—straggling moustache, dribbling cigar, battered hat, dung-buttered boots.

Ole Vet is a lovable old coot, a stereotype that veterinarians cherish and respect just about as much, I would guess, as Julian Bond admires Stepin Fetchit.

I was alive in the days when those celluloid epics were being produced, but I never knew anybody who claimed to have actually seen a living Ole Vet. As far as I know, the Abominable Horse-Doctor never existed.

Even in those days the veterinarian in our town, as in yours, was a professional man who had an office, wore a suit, was a Rotarian, and was proud of his degree of Doctor of Veterinary Medicine. The profession has been a respected and respectable branch of medicine since antiquity. And if I weren't hampered by professional modesty, I would tell you more. Veterinary literature goes back to ancient Greece at least, and in Europe there were prestigious schools of veterinary medicine two hundred years ago—at a time, you will instantly recall, when surgeons were barbers, or vice versa.

Until this century the veterinarian's practice ordinarily included all domestic animals, both great and small. But as the larger beasts were zoned out to the less populated areas, one group of veterinarians specialized mostly in the care of farm animals. Their city colleagues, concerned largely with the care of pets and household creatures, in time came to be called small-animal veterinarians. (That's an awkward title, small-animal veterinarian. And the one that most of them prefer, companion-animal veterinarian, comes no more trippingly to the tongue, though it is more accurately descriptive.)

Today there are hundreds of veterinarians working independently or with other scientists in dozens of fields of research and on government projects affecting nearly every aspect of modern life. But for practicing veterinarians specialization has not gone much beyond what it was half a century ago. While the M.D.s were proliferating into scores of specialties, the D.V.M.s (and V.M.D.s) continued to treat all of the ills that afflict any kind of animal. They were, and for the most part still remain, the only true *general* practitioners in the whole field of medicine.

Unless a veterinarian has unaccountably sprung up in your family, you are unlikely to have any conception of what a veterinarian is expected to do and know and be. You would not take him for a one-man medical facility—which is what he has to be to get through one small morning in one small practice. You see only what you see in the waiting room—the common cat-and-dog problems of bites, hair balls, kidney failure, cuts, worms, arthritis, ear mites, and mange. But there is the surgery, too, where there may well be half a dozen or more animals to be operated on: a cancer to be excised and sent out for a pathological report; a fracture to be repaired with a pin or an intermediary device; a bladder stone to be removed; a case of dysplasia to be corrected; a cataract to be removed; dental work, cleaning, and extractions, for an old dog—or a cat.

While he is in the surgery, the veterinarian must also be responsible for the direction of the whole medical and clerical routine of the establishment. He will be answering calls about animals under treatment at the hospital and getting reports about those being treated at home. He'll have an emergency call or two—a parrot wheezing suddenly, a cat staggering in circles. And in the prevailing quiet the police will arrive with a vicious, convulsing raccoon looped at the end of a dog warden's pole. Is he rabid?

To prepare for this kind of general practice takes more than a smattering of education. The student will spend three or four years in stiff preveterinary study. He will do well, too, or he won't go on to any of the nineteen veterinary schools in the United States. Only *one* out of about seven applicants is accepted. If he does manage to become that one, he will not be encouraged to feel secure. The admissions officers of many of the schools tell the students bluntly that before graduation 10 or 20 percent of those at the bottom of the class will be asked to leave if they do not drop out of their own accord.

For even dedicated students the veterinary curriculum is staggering. Take one example. Anatomy is not the single subject which the M.D. must master. Anatomy for the D.V.M. is the anatomy of the cat, the horse, the hog, the chicken, the cow, the dog, and of a few reptiles, fish, and amphibians. That's *one* subject. There are also (to name only a few others) pathology, reproduction, radiology, nutrition for all these creatures. And, of course, there is chemistry, pharmacology, surgery . . . until strength runs out.

Those who survive four years of veterinary school are permitted to take a written national board examination in which they may be asked to reproduce any segment of any subject they were expected to master in any of the preceding years—the anatomy of the white shark, perhaps. In the state in which he intends to practice, the student takes his practical examination, and there he may have the opportunity to show his dexterity by demonstrating the technique of delivering a turned calf. All this before he may legally advise you on your poodle problem.

These are the vicissitudes. I am not saying that the standards are too high or that the demands are unreasonable, though clearly in this era of exploding knowledge there must be an end to what any one person can be expected to know. What I *am* saying is that the modern veterinarian must, I think, have a broader range of skill and knowledge than a person practicing in any other branch of medicine today.

There used to be a parlor game which involved asking each participant to make a list of what he would most want to have in a small survival kit if he were to be cast, Robinson Crusoe-fashion, on a desolate island. What books, what tools, what utensils, what supplies—and, sometimes, what companion. Generally, the realists reluctantly gave up Shakespeare and the Bible in favor of the world's most complete and detailed book on boat building. And most people, when they were forced to the final-final selection of a companion, abandoned the most admired conversationalist of our time and even the most coveted sex object, and chose instead to have a good doctor with his black bag.

Robinson Crusoeing is rare today. But if you should ever have to make a desperate-situation choice of a companion, I suggest that you try for a seasoned, general-practice veterinarian. Who else among all the medical experts could you find who could treat skin diseases, do a Caesarian section, remove kidney stones, perform a cataract operation, repair a shattered hip, treat a cardiac insufficiency, and handle all of the minor maintenance jobs necessary to keep you alive and functional until you could build the boat and sail home?

In a game of this sort, at least one alert and foresighted man will get a gleam in his eye. Of course there are women veterinarians. Of course. It is true that until recently the obvious frailty and delicacy of women precluded their entering the field. By its very nature the practice of veterinary medicine was either above or below the endowments of women, for clearly no lady had either the stomach to wield a scalpel or the strength to lift a cow. They were excluded from veterinary medicine as they were from people medicine. And from other professions where strength was of paramount importance—law and the ministry, for example. But fortunately, within the last generation or two there has been an enormous increase in the durability and strength of women. There are now more than a token number of female veterinarians in practice (upwards of eight hundred) and there are many more in the making. In 1973 there were 1,002 women among the 5,720 students enrolled in veterinary schools. There is an excellent chance (and I do mean excellent) that before long you will often be saying, "Now, Hector. Stand still. She's not going to hurt you."

I hope it isn't necessary to add that in this book every time you are told to see your veterinarian and ask *him,* the author deplores the conventions of an outmoded grammar as much as you do. But it seemed to me that to use a monstrosity like *her/him* would exasperate even the most militant Ms.

But back to the veterinarian in the making. After he has passed the qualifying examination (and they are so rigorous and the stress is so great that a significant percent of those who take them fail the first time), the young D.V.M. is merely prepared to face the real problems of the real world. I won't burden you with many of them—the large debt that most graduates have dangling from their diplomas, or the poverty period of internship, the lean years when he is getting large experience and small pay as an assistant to an established practitioner. Years later, when ambition and the growing needs of a growing family make him think about establishing his own practice, he may be able to do just that—providing he has paid off his old debts and is able to negotiate a substantial loan from his friendly neighborhood banker. Substantial. In most areas today he will need at least $100,000 to buy the land he needs and build what could be called, in the jargon of the profession, a modest but reasonably complete clinic facility.

His difficulties then—the financial and professional problems of building a practice—of course, need not concern you. But at the same time he will have to cope with the explosive growth of knowledge, technology, and techniques in his field. And that *does* concern you, for the veterinarian who fails to keep abreast of developments for as little as two or three years is slipping into obsolescence. He should not only be reading half a dozen important monthly journals and reviewing perhaps as many basic texts published or revised each year, but he should also be attending regularly scheduled courses which may easily require upwards of fifty hours of classwork during the year.

In time this proliferation of knowledge will have an increasingly important effect on veterinary medicine in general. The cost of setting up a clinic with its essential facilities is so staggeringly high, and each generation of new and improved equipment so expensive that it seems to me the only practical way to make the full range of new, sophisticated equipment fully available is to pool the necessary resources in a general hospital open to all interested, qualified practitioners. In my own community such a facility is now being built and will soon be in operation to serve the needs of those in the surrounding area who want to use it—to the great benefit, certainly, of the veterinarians and their patients.

Another welcome advance is the beginning of specialization which has at last begun to appear in some fields. There are already a few specialists—radiologists, ophthalmologists, dermatologists, toxicologists, orthopedists, and a variety of laboratory specialists—and their numbers are growing. And in some areas these specialists now visit general practitioners on a regular basis for consultation and treatment of difficult problem cases. At long last. May their numbers multiply.

I haven't mentioned geriatrics as an area of specialization. That's not an oversight. It simply doesn't yet exist, though it should. In my opinion specialists in canine geriatrics could serve a great and growing need in an area which has been inadequately explored and for the most part shamefully neglected. We will have veterinary geriatricians. And soon, I hope.

All of this, I know, may seem to be a bit more than you care to know about veterinary medicine and the problems of those who practice it. But it is not more, I think, than you *should* know or *need* to know. The problems which the veterinarian faces inevitably affect the kind of services he can offer his clients, and the solutions which are found will in large part determine the quality, the cost, and the availability of the health care you can provide for your dog.

If many owners are not concerned with the present state and probable future of veterinary medicine as such, they all seem to be troubled with at least one problem: How do you choose a veterinarian?

It is a common, chronic, persistent problem, and like all such enduring questions, it has no short and sufficient answer. So owners continue to ask it of everyone, apparently, including veterinarians. I am asked constantly, generally by people who live at a safe distance from me, presumably because they think that a New England veterinarian will be forthright and honest enough to tell them the truth about veterinarians on the West Coast. That doesn't bother me. What does disturb me is that the man on my left at dinner seems to expect me to give him the inside dope in a sentence or so—two capsules before dessert, as it were.

My own clients are, of course, more perspicacious. They seldom raise the question before the third visit in a very difficult case, and then quite gently: "Gee . . . this is a tough one, isn't it, Doctor? Now, if your dog had a problem like this, who would you take him to?" Everybody knows that the doctor's doctor has to be better than the doctor himself. But unfortunately there is no ultimate wisdom in veterinary medicine, no veterinarian's veterinarian. The M.D. sends his wife and children to a colleague, but the veterinarian treats his own dog.

How do you choose a veterinarian? You choose a veterinarian as you would choose a doctor for yourself. With the same concern, the same thoughtful care, and the same difficulty. And if you have read what has gone before, you will know that is not an arrogant, casual, or flip answer. I know of no easier way, no better way, And I know of no way to avoid all chance of error.

The soundest advice I can give you, I think, is that you make an intelligent effort to get the best out of the veterinarian you already have. You have a dog—a dog who is at least middle-aged—so you surely have a veterinarian. Probably a better veterinarian than you realize. Mark Twain once said that when he was a boy of fourteen, his father was so ignorant that he could hardly stand to have the old man around. But when he got to be twenty-one, he was astonished at how much the old man had learned in seven years. It is possible that as you learn more about old dogs and a bit more about veterinary medicine, you will notice that your veterinarian is appreciably brighter.

Nothing will benefit Hector more than your intelligent and informed cooperation with your veterinarian. Your awareness, your perception, your ability and willingness to follow instructions—these are the essential tools which make it possible for the veterinarian to do his best work. So see him, talk with him, tell him, ask him. Make yourself freely and fully available to help him cope with the special and peculiar difficulties inherent in treating any dumb animal. Interest and concern for Hector are bright and necessary virtues. But an intelligent, genuine willingness to cooperate with the veterinarian is even better medicine.

Above all—and the admonition is so glaringly obvious that I'm almost embarrassed to mention it—above all, don't play games with your veterinarian. You are not there to test him, to compete with him, to stump him with a problem, or to prove that he is not as bright and perceptive as he should be. There are, my lawyer friends tell me, sound reasons to believe that the arms-length, adversary relationship that prevails in court is the surest way to arrive at the truth. That may be. But you are in a veterinarian's office not to settle a dispute, but to get help and advice. The least likely way to get them, surely, is to plump your dog down on the examination table and *defy* the veterinarian to tell you what is wrong with him.

It happens every day. There are people who have an astonishing (and apparently irresistible) inclination to make the veterinarian's job as difficult as they can. They force him to search and probe for clues; they deliberately withhold significant information; they yield background facts as reluctantly as a hostile witness. And they lie. For what reason, I cannot say. If the veterinarian loses this wretched game, who wins?

And yet— Here is an old dog dying in agony on the table in my office. The owner has no clues to offer. No, the dog hasn't been out of the house unattended. No, he couldn't have been raiding a garbage can. No, he just had his regular food. Nothing unusual at all. It just came on him during the night. Can't think of anything. But when we x-ray the dog we find out. He had been fed chicken bones, the whole carcass apparently. We find out, all right. But too late.

And here is an owner explaining that the abdominal swelling of the eleven-year-old Penelope couldn't possibly be a pregnancy. "Couldn't be. She was never out of our sight. Never." She looks pregnant, the veterinarian thinks. But it could be a tumor. Or possibly fluid. It could be, but it wasn't. Beside the man there is his seven-year-old daughter, and she diagnoses the case. "But Daddy, remember how she got out and was gone all night? Remember how we all worried?" The man doesn't look at me, and I can't look at him. You wonder. You have to wonder what goes on in the man's mind, what it was that he was trying to prove. And to whom?

You have a veterinarian. But today we live in a mobile society, and the time may come when, by choice or necessity, you have to find another. You move to a different town, the old veterinarian wears out and closes his office, highways get clogged and gas is rationed, tempers flare—there are dozens of reasons. And you are back again to choosing a veterinarian from the field. How do you go about it?

It's not nearly the ordeal that some people would have you believe it is, and in my biased opinion half of those glooming about the scarcity of good veterinarians have few reasons to complain and still fewer qualifications to make a judgment. Within easy reach of most communities of any consequence there are veterinarians—more than one —and among them there are certainly qualified practitioners with skills and credentials that should satisfy the most demanding owner. It seems to me that a person who with reasonable effort is unable to find a D.V.M. who meets his standards is either myopic or has requirements that are somehow askew. We do, indeed, need more skilled and dedicated veterinarians. We also need more well-informed and perceptive owners—of whom more later.

Suppose you are in a new community. Nobody remains an isolated stranger for long, and most of the people you meet and do business with will be happy to help you with all of the problems of relocation. You'll have a doctor in short order, and the chances are that he will be able to give you very reliable information about the veterinarians in town. The pharmacist will also advise you knowledgeably. With ethical impartiality he'll probably give you the names of two or three veterinarians—all of them well qualified, too, because he fills their prescriptions and is unlikely to suggest those who seldom find the newer drugs useful or depend on outmoded remedies. Your neighbors will have dogs, and presumably their dogs get some medical attention. The real estate agent through whom you bought your house may turn out to be a dog fancier. And down the road somewhere there is sure to be a dog breeder raising the kind of dog you have. He'll be delighted to meet a kindred soul and happy to give you the name of the veterinarian to whom he takes his kennel problems. As you make inquiries, you will find that one or two names are almost always mentioned. And that will tell you something. But beyond that, I hope that you will consider how knowledgeable your informant is, and that you will listen for the specific reasons he gives for recommending a particular veterinarian. All advice is unequal.

The information is certainly not difficult to come by and with a minimal amount of industry you will soon have all you need and more than you can use. The problem is then one of evaluation and generally that can best be done after a visit with one or more of the veterinarians who, from what you have learned about them, seem most likely to fit your needs. You know the kind of information you should have about a veterinarian—and so does he. He's busy, and you can't expect him to sit down for a leisurely chat with you. But unless you come on like a criminal investigator, there is no reason for him to resent your asking pertinent and appropriate questions. Indeed, he is likely to welcome a client who approaches him with candor and intelligent concern. You are quite properly interested in knowing where and when he got his veterinary training and where and how long he has been in practice. You will soon discover what his major interests have been and what fields of study or research he may currently be involved in. You will see what his facilities are and without making a white-glove inspection, you can surely judge the apparent cleanliness and efficiency of the operation. Out of all of this and the general tone of the office you will arrive at a reasonably good estimate of the level of efficiency and proficiency in the place.

Equally important are those intangible qualities which are not seen but rather are heard and perceived. Nobody wears the stripes of his character on his sleeve, but neither is anybody able to conceal himself totally under a white coat. Who knows how one evaluates personal characteristics or how accurate his assessments will turn out to be? But each of us in his own way does make judgments. You should leave the veterinarian's office feeling that the person you have been talking with is thoroughly conscientious, honest, diligent, and ethical. His manner, his way of thinking, his personality should be—for want of a sturdier word—agreeable to you. And most important, you should have a positive feeling of confidence in him, both as a person and as a practitioner.

This sounds, I know, like a list of cardinal virtues from one of McGuffey's *Readers*—and for all I know, it may be. But this I also know: In a relationship of this sort, unless you have a clear and positive feeling about such fundamentals as these, you are off to a bad start. And there's not much that can be done about a relationship that simply fails to jell. It has to do in some obscure way with what we used to call "personal chemistry." Last week, or last year, I'm told, it was called "vibes." If the feeling isn't right, don't ignore it and don't merely hope that it will improve. Go back to your list and try again. You'll be doing everybody a favor—you, Hector, and the veterinarian.

But if you work your way entirely through the list that you have made and still haven't been able to find a veterinarian who satisfies your requirements, then you do have a problem. In fact, I think it is safe to say that *you* have a problem.

Some years ago at a dinner party I was delighted to meet a famous psychoanalyst whose name was in many households and who had written several excellent books, two of which I had read with great interest. He was a stimulating conversationalist and had a most provocative mind. I enjoyed the evening immensely, but the bit I remember most clearly was his shank-of-the-evening summary of a long discussion. "There are many imponderables," he said thoughtfully. "Luck, for example. Look at my case. I have been married five times. I simply have no luck with women. . . ."

It is possible, I suppose, to have the ill luck to encounter a whole series of poorly qualified veterinarians. Or to have standards so high that all but paragons are excluded. Or to land in an area where the practice of veterinary medicine is entirely primitive and substandard. Possible. But remarkable, certainly. A cause for wonder.

You should know, I think, that while you are interviewing veterinarians, you too will be under scrutiny. You are looking for a good veterinarian. And the veterinarian you are talking with is looking for good clients. Surely it will be no surprise to you that the clients he most values are those who have the same qualities you are searching for in a veterinarian, clients who are conscientious, honest, ethical, knowledgeable. . . .

I am not revealing a guarded professional secret when I tell you that veterinarians have their own methods of grading clients. The grading system is often loose and informal. But it is real. And it is important to you. In some large practices the owners' file cards are actually marked with a code or symbol of some sort—A, B, C, D, and yes, a few Es. In a small practice there is less need for a written key; the veterinarian and his assistant can easily carry the records in their heads. But written or remembered, the mark is still there. It is useful for the veterinarian. It gives him a quick help-or-hindrance quotient for the client, and indicates the level of interest and cooperation he can expect. It is also useful when he must make a choice in methods of treating an animal, for often what is done depends at least in part on the knowledge and diligence with which the owner can be expected to follow instructions.

So the mark on your card—not the mark itself, but the attitude it reflects—sometimes and to some degree affects what happens to your dog. More often, I am afraid, than it should. Every veterinarian does the best he possibly can for any animal in his care. He cannot, must not, do less. But nobody, however dedicated, can do his best work if he has to fend off a difficult and disagreeable owner, or if he has to contend with an owner who is plainly indifferent, incompetent, or uncooperative. He will try his best. Of course he will. But he can't possibly avoid the realization that his efforts are certain to be less effective than they might have been with the willing and intelligent cooperation of the owner. It is equally true that the veterinarian working with the wholehearted support of a capable owner often surpasses his own best expectations. With the same effort he achieves more. Not sometimes, but often. I think that it is wrong that what happens to an animal should in any way depend on his owner's attitude or relationship to the veterinarian. But inevitably and unavoidably, it does. You should know that. And you should be concerned about where you stand on your veterinarian's list.

Obviously, I can't tell you how *the* veterinarian arrives at his estimates of his clients. But I have recently had occasion to review my own list, and I *can* give you a summary of what one group of clients looks like to one veterinarian. They are, I suspect, a more diversified group than you would find in many practices. They differ widely in economic, social, and ethnic backgrounds, and they live in the city, suburbs, towns, and so-called rural areas around about. I would guess they are somewhat above *average*—however you choose to define that—and if they are typical of anything, it is only that they are typical southern New Englanders who have companion animals. As a whole, you will see, they are good people, and I wouldn't swap them off for any practice that I know of. As a whole. There are a few who still need improvement.

Ten percent of the people in my practice are straight-A clients. They are what I have been telling you that a client *should* be. They are thoughtful, concerned, cooperative owners who care for their pets intelligently and who have the sense and foresight never to let a minor problem escalate into a major one before they seek help. They bring their animals in for checkups, they phone for an opinion when a puzzling problem arises, they are knowledgeable enough not to cry wolf at the appearance of a trivial symptom. When they come to the office, they are prepared to describe the problem clearly and fully, and to answer questions directly and honestly. While the examination is going on, they don't regale me with tales of their vacation adventures, and they don't ask urgently what I think should be done about Grandpa's gout—which never seems to improve. They ask questions when they need to—and hear answers. When the problems are difficult, they don't complicate them by proposing a dozen impossible solutions. They make decisions without vacillating from yes to no to maybe yes. When they feel that they haven't enough knowledge to choose wisely between alternatives, they say so. In the crunch they are willing to say, "I don't know what to tell you. I want you to treat Hector exactly the way you would treat your own dog." And I do. They are great clients. May they prosper and multiply.

The B group is twice as large—perhaps 20 percent—and if they are not among the very best, they are still very good indeed. They have all the virtues—well, almost all—and I love them as much as the A group—well, almost. They are no less concerned, but they are not quite as alert and well informed. They tend to drift off into extraneous matters when we are discussing a problem, to raise what-if questions about unlikely complications, to expect prophetic assurances and prognostications. They are dedicated but not dextrous, cooperative but unsure and sometimes inept. But they are fine folk. Their attitude is excellent, their intentions always good, and many of them are no more than one dog away from an A rating.

Half of my practice is with the C group. An average client is an average client, agreeable and good-hearted, troubled and troublesome. She is genuinely concerned about little old Penelope, but often in a kind of dispassionate, once-removed way: "She's not much of a dog, but the kids kept pestering us. With my husband away so much . . . I guess the kids would miss her." They are the kind of people who hope that things will work out for the best—or at least won't get worse. But often they hope and procrastinate until things do get worse. They are that way with almost everything. By the time the house is painted the siding has begun to rot, the car limps along until it stops on the road, and there is a red, bare patch the size of a silver dollar on Penelope's back before the veterinarian is asked to look at it. When he does bring the dog to the office, it takes the C client a long time to get around to explaining the symptoms as he sees them—and even longer to review the remarkable series of coincidences that prevented his getting there sooner. But he knows that he has bungled this one, and he'll make a conscientious effort to make up for it. The veterinarian does the best he can for the dog—and for the client. He urges. He complains. The next time, he hopes . . . And often it works. The C client is not a bad guy, really. But he does take a lot of time. And patience. And help.

The 15 percent who fall into the D category—the barely passing grade—are a strange lot of difficult and disagreeable people. Almost invariably they are extremely something-or-other. They are never reasonably, or generally, or mildly anything. Some profess—indeed they insist—that they love their dogs more than anything in this world. More than their husbands, more than their wives, and, yes (I have had them tell me), more than their children. And sometimes I am tempted to believe them. Their knowledge is limited and their imagination vast. A woman once called me at three o'clock in the morning—they are all insomniacs with enormous telephone bills—to tell me that her dog had just fallen off the sofa and ruptured his appendix. Another made a scene in the office because I refused to interrupt a Caesarian section to look at her dog's lame leg. (He did have a slight limp. I had noticed it a month or so earlier, but she had discovered it only that morning.)

These demanding, determined, disruptive people can make a shambles of any day. I once had a client who was a plague in my office for years, particularly to the staff and the young veterinarians. She regularly began her attack by making small unpleasantries with the receptionist when she called to negotiate an appointment. She arrived armed with complaints—complaints about the animals and the people in the waiting room, about the examination, the instructions, the medication, the bill. And after she left, she phoned in criticisms she had forgotten to deliver in person. Eventually I was the only person in the office who could abide her, and finally I wore thin. "Mrs. Out-of-the-wrong-side-of-the-bed," I said one day, "we have never been able to do *anything* that pleased you. Why do you keep coming back?" "Don't think I haven't tried others," she snapped. "I have. They're worse!" Poor woman. At last she deceased and desisted.

Among this group there are others who come to the veterinarian only as a last resort, only to divest themselves of problems they haven't been able to get rid of any other way. A man brings in his dog with a lacerated foot, an old wound that has become badly infected. "It happened last night," the man says blandly. I look at him. "Last night," he repeats stoutly. Does he think I am an idiot? But the dog is hurting, and there is nothing to do but to start cleaning up the old wound.

Or there is a night emergency call. "My old Boxer is having convulsions. He's thrashing all over the room and foaming at the mouth." How long has that been going on? "Oh, for two or three hours, I guess." I would have like to have said, "Well, if you let it go on for two or three hours, why not wait and bring him in next week?" Instead I urged the man to rush the dog to my office and told him I would meet him there. Two hours later he arrived. It was garbage poisoning: stomach pump, intravenous fluids, shock treatment. But all too late.

And always there is the man-in-a-hurry. Many of them. He brings in a tottering old dog and hardly has time to wait while we examine him. When we tell him that the neglected animal is in a near-hopeless condition, he pauses at the door. "Well, fix him up, Doc." As though he were dropping his wife's vacuum cleaner off at the repair shop. Is there any hope for such people?

And finally (if you haven't been keeping a running total), there is the bottom 5 percent—the Terribles. There is little that I can say *for* them, and the best that can be said *about* them is that they are few. They have neither knowledge nor compassion and they are belligerently confident of their competence in all circumstances. They are a menace to their dogs and an affliction to veterinarians.

Nothing that can be done wrong escapes them. If they are willing to consult a veterinarian at all—and I know, of course, that many, if not most, people of this sort never get inside a veterinarian's office—they delay until even a minor problem has grown into a disaster. When they do appear, they tell the veterinarian what his diagnosis should be, why the treatment he proposes is wrong, how the condition can be cured overnight—and cheaply. Once, when I told a man that his crippled dog had a form of arthritis that seemed worse than it actually was and that the dog could be successfully treated, he said, "Oh. Better give him the black bottle, Doc." I had never heard the expression before, and it took me a moment to realize what the man was saying. When I did, I asked him to leave. But I kept the dog.

These people are all expert at home medication. Their heads are full of old wives' tales and folk tortures, and every one of them seems to keep a file of fads and miracle cures that the medical profession hasn't had the wit to discover. With the help of Uncle Ezra, who is a good butcher and used to own a dog, they are prepared to treat any condition. With superstition and stump water (and sometimes with the reckless use of drugs they know nothing about) they do an immense amount of damage to defenseless animals.

There are not many such owners, fortunately, but they constitute a problem out of proportion to their number. Veterinarians have an obligation to treat all animals in need of their services, and they don't lightly disregard that duty even when the person at the other end of the leash is energetically objectionable. Some veterinarians, I believe, feel that under circumstances of extreme provocation they have an inalienable right to "throw the bum out." And occasionally they do that. But rarely. In thirty years of practice I have actually thrown only two clients out of my office. Perhaps there should have been more. But bouncing a few individuals out of the office is no solution to the larger problem. Instead, we have to get these people *into* the veterinarians' offices, we have to persuade them to get professional treatment for their animals when they need it, and—at the very least—we have to find a way to prevent them from doing the kind of harm they are capable of. How that is to be done, I don't know. But somehow it *must* be done.

You are looking for a good veterinarian. You need one. And you'll find one with less difficulty than you think. But that is not all you need. What I am saying here is that while you are looking for a veterinarian, you should also be looking at yourself. What you are really looking for is a way for you and your veterinarian to work effectively together to help each other help old Hector.

VIII
The Ills of Age

All old dogs have problems. The problems of age. Old dogs *do* run down, wear down, and break down with a variety of ills. And it is sensible and proper for you to want to know something about the difficulties your dog is likely to have as he grows older. You do want to know what the common problems are. You also want to know what causes them, when to expect them, what can be done to prevent or ameliorate them. And you should know.

But you should also be cautioned that any discussion of the ailments your dog *may* get is also necessarily a discussion of a host of ailments your dog won't get. Any list, even though it is rigorously confined to problems that occur frequently—as this one is—is apt to seem alarmingly long. It *could* be read as a threatening inventory of impending calamities. And it could, I suppose, induce a kind of vicarious hypochondria in a suggestible owner and lead him to see "symptoms" where none exist. But it won't, I trust. You have been forewarned, and you should be forearmed.

There is another danger. The problems here are

described in terms of their symptoms, for obviously it is only by their signs and symptoms that you will recognize them.

Medical dictionaries, professors and other respected authorities once made much ado about the difference between a *sign* and a *symptom*. They insisted that the designation *symptom* was correctly used only when it referred to a *subjective* indication of disease which led to complaints by the patient, and that the word *sign* was properly applied only to *objective* physical evidence which could be observed by someone other than the patient. Arguments about the usage of these terms sometimes reached the intensity of theological disputes, and those who were so inclined could spend happy hours discussing the semantic subtleties of such seemingly self-contradictory terms as *subjective sign* and *objective symptom*.

Niceties had their time and may still have their places—but not, I think, in an antitechnical book about old dogs. Here and there sticklers continue to stickle, but even the lexicographers seem to have abandoned the purists. *Webster*'s *New International Dictionary, Second Edition, Unabridged* (1938) defines *symptom* as: "1. *Med.* Any perceptible change in the body or its functions, either subjective or objective, which indicates disease, or the kind or phases of disease . . ." And the Random House *American College Dictionary* (1964) says that the word means: "2. *Pathol.* a phenomenon that arises from and accompanies a particular disease or disorder and serves as an indication of it."

I am firmly permissive about the use of these words. Your dog may have either a sign or a symptom, as he pleases. I am satisfied with either—so long as it leads me to a sound diagnosis.

Symptoms are descriptive tools. You already know—and you will undoubtedly be told again—that a symptom is a slippery thing, and that the same sign may point to one condition in one context and to quite a different one in another. What you are told about signs here is simply to alert you to the possibility that a particular condition may exist, not to lead you to think that you are qualified to make a diagnosis and to decide on the basis of the evidence that you have that it *does* exist. Once again—and unnecessarily, I hope—let me say that diagnosis is the veterinarian's responsibility. Not yours. And for him—with all of the facilities available to him, all of the skill and experience that he has accumulated, all of his five senses and the intuitive sixth as well—it is difficult enough.

It is difficult because signs are always obscure and obvious, confused and clear, unmistakable and contradictory. They point everywhere and nowhere and by their very nature often seem to be contrived to mislead the unwary. And in interpreting them, logic and intelligence alone are not infallible guides. H. L. Mencken might well have been speaking of the pitfalls in making a diagnosis—but wasn't—when he said, "For every problem there is a solution—simple, neat, and wrong."

In our office we have a name for the brilliantly deductive diagnosis based on one or two clear and obvious symptoms. It is called the Zebra Diagnosis.

Many years ago, when wisdom was rare and valuable (the story goes) the council of wise men was gathered one day in the Thinkers' Chamber high in the tower of the king's castle somewhere in merrie medieval Europe. While they were deep in thought grappling with profound problems of state, they heard a sudden clatter of hoof beats in the courtyard below.

"Hark," said the Elder Councillor. "What can that be?"

The members sat and pondered.

"Animals," said one thinker.

"In the courtyard," said another.

"Hoofed animals," said a third.

"And many of them," added still another.

And the wisest of all of them, one renowned for his

reasoning powers, summarized the evidence. "Ah, yes. It is quite clear. A herd of zebras has strayed into the courtyard."

And the Council turned again to the consideration of more difficult matters. Only the page by the window was uneasy. He could see the troop of armed horsemen below.

Nevertheless, learned councillors are not to be scorned. Not long ago we had in the clinic a fine, exquisitely groomed kennel dog who had an acutely painful and destructive condition that seemed to be centered somewhere behind the right eye. We looked, we examined, we probed, we peered with lights, we x-rayed the animal's head, we used every diagnostic device we could think of—and still we were unable to determine the cause. In what may have been our seventh session one of us mused, "It might be . . . if it had worked up through the lip and face—it is just possible that the problem *could* be a porcupine quill." "Zebra!" we all said. "A pampered city dog, a kennel dog like that?" But later I *did* call the owner and ask sheepishly, "Your dog has never been where he could have been quilled by a porcupine, has he?" "Yes. Yes, he has. Last summer in Vermont. But we had them all removed, of course."

All but one. There *were* zebras in the courtyard that time.

Alexander Pope's half-couplet, "A little learning is a dangerous thing," is a half-truth that itself is a dangerous thing. For a century it has been conveniently misquoted by self-styled experts—" A little *knowledge* is a dangerous thing"—and used mainly to blackjack people who are humble enough to admit that they don't know *everything* about a particular subject. Anything—much or little —that is misused is dangerous. And whatever the poets say, I can tell you that any veterinarian would rather deal with an owner who knows *something* about the problem than with one who knows nothing about it.

There are, of course, clients who don't *want* to hear what is happening to their dogs. "Don't tell me more than I need to know," they say. Or "Don't bother to explain the details, Doc. Just fix him up the best you can." But when clients have that attitude it is hard to "fix him up" and impossible to "do the best you can." And so, both as a matter of principle and because it makes my job easier, I tell them what the problems are. I tell them first what I think they must know if they are to be of any help, and sometimes—time permitting—I try to give them the background information that they *ought* to have. If these explanations don't invariably interest or comfort the owners, they do, I think, benefit their dogs.

Here then, in briefest form, is the substance of some of the background discussions of some of the common difficulties that old dogs encounter. The common ills and infirmities. There are no once-in-a-great-while rarities among them and no believe-it-or-not zebra diagnoses. The descriptions are abbreviated, stripped of clinical details, and as free of jargon as I can make them. There is not enough information, I hope, to make you feel that you are competent either to diagnose your dog's condition or to treat it yourself. But there should be enough here to encourage you to get professional help at a time when it can be most effective and to enable you to work more knowledgeably with your veterinarian when your dog needs his help.

Heart Problems

. . . and the conditions associated with them, worry owners more than any others—mainly, I suppose, because they are the greatest single cause of death among human beings. Even though heart diseases do not account for as high a proportion of fatalities in dogs, nothing so alarms a client as a diagnosis which suggests any kind of heart condition. Heart disease does take its toll of dogs, but contrary to what most people fear, the discovery of a weakness or irregularity in the function of the heart is not tantamount to a death sentence.

It is always difficult to convince owners that a heart fault of any kind does not spell imminent disaster, and for years Wendy has been my most useful persuader. Wendy bore two lifelong handicaps, neither of which appeared to distress him. One was his name. He had the misfortune to arrive in a politically active family in the midst of an exciting presidential campaign, and he was disastrously named Wendell Willkie. Since nobody could bring himself to call a bustling Cocker Spaniel *Wendell,* and since I was unable to persuade his owners that calling him *Willkie* would at least avoid scandalous gossip, he manfully lived all his life with the name *Wendy.*

The second problem was his heart. I first examined him when he was six weeks old. Instead of a heartbeat there was the sound of a large, juicy orange being stepped on hard. I had to tell the owners that though he appeared to be an unusually busy, active pup, he had a heart that was nearly useless. I could only suggest that they let him enjoy life while he could and warn them to be prepared for the worst at any time. They had ample time to prepare themselves. Though Wendy never had a single normal heartbeat in his life, for fourteen years (at first to my embarrassment and then to my amazement and delight) he shared the unusually active life of his owners—including their annual hiking, canoeing, and (so help me) mountain-climbing vacations. And his heart never did give out. It was an inoperable cancer that finally ended his fun.

There are, of course, few Wendys. But many dogs survive for years with defective hearts. Pathologists who have examined the hearts of thousands of dogs have found evidence of disease conditions present in nearly 75 percent of those who are seven years old or older. And that is long before a dog usually shows any of the symptoms of the common problems—inflammation of the heart muscle itself or of its surface, weakness and insufficiency, or valve trouble.

A dog's heart has capabilities well beyond the demands usually made on it, sufficient reserve strength and capacity to function well under the most extreme conditions of stress. Even after aging has reduced its efficiency substantially, it is still able to do its work remarkably well. But in time muscular deterioration does reach a point where the heart is unable to respond to the peak demands made on it—prolonged exertion or a sudden failure of another organ. The dog begins to show such symptoms as shortness of breath, general fatigue and sluggishness, easy tiring during moderate activity, and a cough, particularly after exercise.

This weakness—it is called *cardiac insufficiency*—is treatable, and the dog can generally be greatly helped if you are alert to the symptoms and report them to your veterinarian before the process has gone too far. In addition to the usual stethoscope examination, he will often find it necessary to further check his findings with an electrocardiogram and possibly with a chest x-ray. If the latter is necessary, the dog will probably have to be left with the veterinarian for a day or overnight since it is difficult to position the dog properly for pictures unless he is under anesthesia.

If treatment is begun in time, medication—which may include a carefully regulated dosage of a derivative of digitalis or one of several other medicaments—is generally effective in controlling the condition. Once begun, the medication usually must be continued on a fixed and regular schedule. It is not, however, difficult to establish such a routine, and owners treating their dogs at home sometimes tell me that if they do not appear with the medicine promptly at the established time, their dogs often come to remind them of the oversight. With treatment a dog may live a near-normal life for years. But untreated, cardiac insufficiency becomes progressively worse. The circulation of the blood is reduced so severely and the shortage of oxygen becomes so acute that the dog begins to pant even when he is at rest. The tragic end is that unless he gets help, the dog will eventually die of what amounts to slow asphyxiation.

Leaking valves are not at all uncommon in dogs. They are sometimes congenital—as in Wendy's case—but what causes them to develop in older dogs has not been established. They do, of course, decrease the efficiency of the heart and when the action of the valve falls below a certain level of effectiveness the dog can no longer survive. But the capability of the heart is such that it is easily able to compensate for a considerable malfunctioning of the valves. Only in very severe cases does a valve condition immediately threaten a dog's life. Indeed—as witness Wendy again—a dog may be able to live a long, normally active life in spite of a leaky valve.

The heart does not function alone but in intimate relation to all of the organs of the body, and both the symptoms and effects of heart problems are seen in many areas. The heart and lungs are close, not only geographically but also in their functions. If the heart does not pump sufficient blood to the lungs, a shortage of oxygen—*anoxia*—develops. More blood is then poured into the lungs to correct this condition, and if the lungs are unable to release the wastes rapidly enough, carbon dioxide and fluid accumulate to excessive levels and cause the cough which is a characteristic symptom of the heart patient. When the heart condition is treated, the cough is generally alleviated or eliminated.

As the dog grows older, the aging process affects all parts of the body. The elasticity of the lungs and of the arterial system begins to disappear. The hardening of the arteries increases the load on the heart and compounds the problem of circulating blood to all parts of the body. If the kidneys are inadequately supplied, they begin to fail to filter the waste products from the system. If the liver is deprived, it cannot detoxify the blood adequately and all of the tissues of the body will be affected to some degree. Eventually somewhere in the body some part will fail to function at even a minimal level. The operation of the heart cannot forever be maintained and supported by medication. But timely treatment of a weakening heart can and does provide the support which makes it possible for it to continue its crucial function long after it would otherwise have failed.

Strokes

. . . are caused by the rupture of a blood vessel in the brain. Why that happens when it happens is still not well understood, and we are unable to account for the fact that strokes often occur in dogs that appear to be normal and in good health. Usually the symptoms appear suddenly and without warning. At first the dog seems to be deeply depressed and begins to show signs of severe apprehension. Often this is followed by a compulsion to circle continuously, always in a single direction, either to the left or to the right. Generally the eyes are affected too. One pupil is often noticeably larger than the other and in many cases the eyes twitch rapidly from side to side. This is called *nystagmus*.

The severity depends upon the size of the brain area affected, but with dogs strokes are generally not as incapacitating as they are with human beings. The muscles of one area may be affected slightly or severely, but the dog is almost never generally paralyzed. He seldom loses his voice, but the tone and quality of the sound may be noticeably changed. A dog's recovery from a stroke is quicker, more common, and generally more complete than it is with a person. Nor does the fact that a dog has had a stroke appreciably increase the likelihood of another.

A stroke is, of course, reason to call your veterinarian at any hour. Depending on the severity of the symptoms, he will want to see the dog either instantly or soon for a thorough examination and perhaps a laboratory workup. He may be able to prescribe medication to relieve the symptoms—often it is impossible to get the dog to sleep or even to lie down—and to advise you about diet and the problems of feeding that may have arisen. Beyond that, it is largely a matter of waiting to see if the body can repair the damage—and if it can, how well. Fortunately, that often takes less time than you would expect. Many times I have seen a dramatic improvement within a few days.

There are other conditions which somewhat resemble the effects of a slight stroke in a person but which, in a dog, are caused by a failure somewhere in the nervous system. One such problem is similar to a partial facial paralysis in a person. In dogs the effects are generally seen on one side only—a sagging of the lip, drooling, a drooping of the lower eyelid. The most disturbing result of this kind of local paralysis is that it often makes eating and drinking a great problem for the dog. But he learns in time to live with the difficulty, and very gradually—often over a period of months—some improvement usually takes place.

Any damage to a nerve or any blocking of the impulses which it carries affects the tissues of the area which it serves. If a nerve is severed before it enters a group of muscles—or if it fails to function for any reason—the muscles become inactive and in time they shrink and atrophy. The muscles on the top of the head are commonly so affected, producing the bulging so-called "bump of knowledge" as they become shorter and thicker. Shoulder muscles are also subject to this loss of nerve connections. When that happens, however, other muscles and nerves are often used to compensate for the loss and the old dog may be able to get around surprisingly well with the use of the alternate set. A nerve serving the intestines is sometimes damaged and causes a sluggish or inactive bowel, a condition which is difficult to treat or even to diagnose. And severe damage to any of the major nerve connections to the eyes can cause a baffling total or partial blindness.

All of these conditions are caused by local failures in parts of the nervous system. They are not the result of a *cerebral accident,* a stroke.

Cancer

. . . remains the most baffling and destructive of diseases, a chronic and invasive growth which can and does occur in almost any part of the body. It takes an enormous and growing toll of lives—among dogs as it does among people —and the intensive effort to unravel the cause-cure complexities of this greatest of all remaining scourges has rightly become the sole objective of thousands of medical scientists and others in related fields. Every clue, however insignificant it may seem, is being investigated. It is worth saying—and more than parenthetically—that veterinary medicine has had, and undoubtedly will continue to have, a crucial part in the race to find the solution to this intricate puzzle on which the lives of millions of people depend.

There is no longer any need to talk about the ravages of cancer. It is more profitable and productive during this period before the riddle is fully and finally solved—this *brief* period, most scientists now believe—to stress the fact that even today we are no longer helpless and hopeless victims of the disease.

Everybody knows that cancer can kill. That is true. But so great is the fear inspired by the word—a term which includes a great number of related diseases—that people tend to believe that *all* cancers kill. And that is *not* true. *Some* do. But many types of cancer *can* be cured and *are being* cured. If a cancer is discovered in time and if it can be completely removed before it has sent out colonies, it will not return to the original site and it will not reappear elsewhere in the body. That is a *cure.* And that has been done thousands and thousands of times.

Because of the fear and misinformation associated with the very word *cancer,* many veterinarians, like most physicians, are reluctant to use the term. They prefer to call a cancer a tumor—which is what it is. Not all tumors are cancerous, of course. Most, in fact, are not. Tumors are classified in two major groups: *benign tumors* which are usually self-contained and often self-limiting; and *malignant tumors* which proliferate beyond the normal limits of growth, invade and destroy adjacent tissue, and sometimes set up colonies elsewhere in the body. The significant difference between the two is that the cancerous, malignant growths have somehow escaped from the controls which regulate normal growth and so are able to increase indefinitely. The search for the cause of that uncontrollable growth is the search for the cause and cure of cancer.

There are many different types of cancer and medical scientists have devised a precise nomenclature to describe them. For example, a *carcinoma* is a cancer arising in the epithelium, the tissue which forms the skin and lines the organs which have openings outside the body. A *sarcoma* is one which grows in the so-called connective tissues such as the bones, muscles, and fatty tissue. These terms can be combined with other descriptive terms to form names which describe a particular growth still more specifically.

More important to the layman than these technical classifications are the differences in growth patterns which occur in the different types of cancer. Because they proliferate rapidly either in the area in which they originate or in colonies elsewhere in the body, some cancers pose an immediate threat to life which can be eliminated only by their prompt and complete surgical removal from the body. Others are, as the pathologists say, *locally* invasive but are not apt to be *metastatic*—which means that they will continue to grow at the point of origin but are not likely to spread through the body. Still others, for reasons that are even less well understood, grow erratically, sometimes becoming quiescent for a while or even regressing, and then suddenly entering a new period of active growth at a later time.

The important thing for you to remember is that there is no possible way for you to distinguish between the various types of cancer or to determine the course which any particular one will take. The only prudent and sensible thing you can do is to report *any* unusual or suspicious growth your dog develops to your veterinarian as soon as you discover it. In some instances he may by examining it be able to identify it with some certainty. Veterinarians have a respectable record for accuracy in this area. But no matter how experienced a practitioner may be, in many cases only a pathologist's examination will firmly and finally establish a diagnosis. Often your veterinarian will explain to you that even though the lesion does not appear to be malignant, he feels that it is wiser to remove the growth immediately on the very real chance that the pathologist's report will later show that it was indeed dangerous.

How early a cancer is detected and where it is located are both critically important in determining the procedure which the veterinarian can use. Cancers that appear as growths on exposed parts of the body are generally discovered early, and since they can be excised relatively easily and completely, the chances of eliminating them permanently are comparatively good. Internal cancers are likely to be diagnosed much later and consequently they have often had time to invade one or more of the vital organs. In an old dog the lungs are often invaded by these colonies, and before undertaking an operation for some types of cancer, the veterinarian will often take a chest x-ray after the dog has been anesthetized. If there are lesions of the lungs, the operation is generally not performed.

In the early stages, a dog with lung cancer sometimes does not appear to be in serious difficulty, and some owners elect to keep him until the symptoms do become severe. That seems to me to be a questionable kindness. It is a sad and difficult thing to live with a dog knowing that he has a malignancy which must inevitably destroy him in a short time. And to wait week after week to decide when he should be released from his suffering, must, it seems to me, be intolerably traumatic for everybody in the family. It is kinder and wiser, I believe, not to let the dog come out of the anesthetic at the time the x-ray shows a cancer from which he cannot recover.

But happily many internal cancers—even very large ones—can be removed from old dogs with remarkably good results. So good, in fact, that unless the case is plainly hopeless, I usually urge the owner to let me at least attempt to correct the problem. Even when the dog is very old. Most people agree that an operation that adds six good months to an old dog's life is well worth the effort. In many cases that can easily be achieved. And often the time bonus is much larger, sometimes running into years.

Once in a while—not often, but it does happen occasionally—when an owner brings in a dog with an enormously distended abdomen, I have the great pleasure of telling him that his dog has *only* a cancer of the spleen, that both the cancer and the expendable organ can be removed and that within a matter of days he will once again have a perfectly sound dog. (But if splenic tumors of this sort are not removed, they often grow uncontrollably until suddenly they rupture and cause death in a matter of minutes.) The largest tumor I have ever removed—largest in proportion to the size of the dog—came from a very old dog whose abdomen was stretched beyond what it would have been had she been ready to have a record litter of pups. Her problem was not pups—she was far past that age—but a cancerous ovary which turned out to be larger than her head. She tolerated the anesthetic well, recovered quickly, and lived an active, girlish life for well over a year after the operation.

Unspayed females have a high incidence of tumors in the mammary area. Usually they do not spread through the system, but if they are not removed surgically, they often grow to massive size, rupture, and become infected. They tend to grow during heat periods or at the culmination of a false pregnancy and to remain quiet or even to regress slightly between the periods. But with each heat they are likely to grow beyond their previous size and eventually to shorten the dog's life. Spayed bitches do live longer, and one of the reasons is that they escape this problem.

Surgical removal is the only certain cure we have for cancer. But not all cancers must be, should be, or can be removed. Sometimes—and this is particularly true of old dogs—a cancer will develop for a time and then stop growing altogether. In such cases the veterinarian may elect not to operate until and unless the cancer enters another period of growth. Other cancers remain small and are so mildly invasive that they pose no threat to the dog's life. Still others grow so slowly that when they develop in a very old dog there is little likelihood that they will become a real danger during his remaining years.

Some types of cancer metastasize so quickly that even when the primary tumor is detected very early, there is still a strong probability that cancerous colonies have been established elsewhere in the body. Often the veterinarian will operate in the hope that he is intervening in time or that, at worst, he will be able to prolong the dog's life significantly. But if an operation is to be fully successful, every bit of malignant tissue must be removed. When the cancer is embedded in a vital organ, that cannot be done. The cancer is, we say, inoperable, and all that can be done is to keep the dog free of pain as long as that can be done and to release him from his suffering before it becomes intolerable.

There are a few things that I hope every owner will believe and remember. Though it is true that some cancers are quick and savage killers, it is equally true today that many cancers—if, indeed, not *most*—can be cured (totally removed and permanently eliminated) or their growth can be slowed and their effects appreciably postponed by early detection and timely intervention. But even more important than that, I hope that owners also realize that the percentage of cures could and *should* be much higher than it actually is. Every year thousands of dogs who could have been saved die because of their owners' fears and misconceptions—because they are afraid that the veterinarian will find that the growth they have seen developing *is* cancerous, because they mistakenly believe that cancer is inevitably fatal, because they foolishly postpone the day of truth until the opportunity to save the dog's life has been tragically, needlessly lost. They worry while their dogs die. Of cancer, we say. It would be more accurate to report that the dogs died of their owners' *fear* of cancer.

Benign Growths and Tumors

. . . can and do appear at any time, in many forms, and on almost any part of any dog's body. Like cancerous growths, their causes are unknown and their development is often unpredictable. Generally they are not life-threatening in themselves since they are self-contained and do not invade and destroy other tissue. But often they must be removed either because they become so large and obstructive that they interfere with the function of some organ or because they cannot be easily and certainly identified as nonmalignant. And unhappily, old dogs are prone to growths of this sort.

Perhaps the most common of the nuisance variety

are *warts.* They can appear almost anywhere on the body, most frequently on the feet or on the tops of the toes, sometimes on the face and nose or along the back. They usually remain insignificantly small, and unless they become uncommonly large or so numerous that they are unsightly, there is seldom any need to have them removed surgically. Occasionally, however, if they become such an annoyance to the dog that he persists in licking or biting them, it becomes a kindness to both the dog and his owner to have them removed.

Another common growth in this category is the *sebaceous cyst,* a lump of a waxy substance which forms in a small gland under the skin. These, too, are generally no more than a nuisance to the dog and a mild inconvenience to the groomer. But now and then one will continue to grow until it becomes ugly and protruding. And occasionally—but only occasionally—a dog will develop dozens of these cysts along his back. In such cases they must be removed—and a tedious chore it is, because unless they are removed cleanly and with surgical precision, they will return.

Fatty tumors are also common in old dogs—in fat old dogs, for they seldom occur in dogs that are not overweight. After they have reached a modest size, they generally stop growing and remain unchanged for the rest of the dog's life. Unless they are conspicuous and ugly, there is no need to bother with them. But lesions which grow where they obstruct movement—on an elbow where the growth may rub against the body, for example—obviously must be removed so that the dog can move comfortably.

Tumors may also grow in or on almost any of the organs. Those that remain small generally cause no difficulties. Indeed, they often go undetected for years and are discovered only in the course of an examination necessary for some unrelated condition. But if they continue to grow—as many of them do—they may become so large that they obstruct an organ and interfere with its function. Depending on its location, such a tumor can cause a great variety of symptoms which are often difficult to interpret. A tumor of the stomach may cause a dog to become a chronic vomiter. In the lower intestine, it may cause a kind of stubborn diarrhea which cannot be relieved by any change in diet. A large tumor of the prostate can exert pressure against the colon and create severe constipation.

Internal tumors may show in x-ray pictures, but often they do not. Sometimes it is necessary for the veterinarian to do an exploratory operation solely on the basis of the symptoms and such other evidence as he can discover. Once it has been established that a tumor is in fact the cause of a malfunction, it can often be removed without danger and the dog completely and permanently relieved of his difficulties.

Benign tumors are generally obstructive rather than destructive. But for the owner the problem is that he has no way of knowing whether a growth is harmlessly benign or destructively malignant. To decide that it is or is not malignant because it *looks* dangerous or does not look dangerous is simply to gamble. You have to be foolish to risk your dog's life in a blind game of chance. A sensible person will let his veterinarian—and a pathologist—make a proper diagnosis.

The Kidneys

. . . are a complex and delicately balanced filtration system so ingeniously contrived and so marvelously adapted to their purpose that for the lifetime of the dog they can function ceaselessly and without rest performing the intricate miracle of cleansing the blood and ridding the body of toxic wastes.

They can—and sometimes they do. Like the heart, the kidneys are programmed to handle far more work than the body normally requires. When the dog is young, each kidney has some 400,000 microscopic filtering units, enough to perform the usual tasks several times over. But in time many of these units are broken down or destroyed by massive overloads of poisons produced by disease, infections, and toxic substances—or perhaps they simply wear out. In an old dog the kidneys are often functioning with no more than 20 or 25 percent of the units still strong and healthy. When that happens, the margin of safety has been lost and the kidneys are vulnerable to sudden and unusual stress. In many old dogs they are the weakest link in the system of interdependent functions and they are often the first to fail.

The function of the kidneys can be impaired by a great variety of conditions throughout the body. If the heart is unable to maintain sufficient pressure to pump 10 or 20 percent of the blood through the kidneys in a continuous flow, they will be unable to keep up with the task of removing impurities from the bloodstream. They can then be overwhelmed by poisonous substances or overburdened by the toxins produced by chronic disease or massive infections. And if the blood is inadequately purified, all the tissues of the body are affected.

The symptoms of kidney problems can be as varied as their causes. With conditions that build up slowly, they are often subtle, almost imperceptible. The old dog may gradually begin to seem a little logy and unresponsive. He doesn't seem to be hurting anywhere, but a bit later he may show signs of discomfort if you apply a little pressure on each side of the back behind the ribs. The first clear and obvious symptom will probably be his need to urinate more frequently, and that, in turn, will sharply increase his desire for fluids. As the condition grows worse, he will drink more and more. Often a medium-sized dog—of forty pounds, say—will drink as much as a gallon of water a day, and his abdomen will become greatly distended. By this time there is usually some blood in the urine, though for a time it may look normal. As the bleeding increases the urine will become rusty-colored or even red.

When the kidney function is *suddenly* impaired or the condition is one that develops rapidly, the symptoms are more evident, sometimes dramatically severe. The dog will vomit and become desperately sick. His respiration will be rapid, he will have severe diarrhea, and sometimes his breath may even smell of urine. Needless to say, these are the signs of a panic-button problem. If the dog's life is to be saved, you will have to get him to the veterinarian immediately so that he can be put under round-the-clock intensive care.

These diseases of sudden onset are not uncommon with old dogs. They are acute and dangerous, and if they are not treated immediately, they can be fatal. But they are not necessarily disastrous. If they are discovered in time and recognized as emergencies, they can usually be treated successfully.

Among the more gradual, progressive diseases is *nephritis*—or, more fully, *interstitial nephritis*—an inflammation of the kidneys. It generally runs a long, slow course. The symptoms tend to be mild at the beginning, but as the condition worsens the dog may seem to be unsteady on his feet. Later he will begin to stagger and fall down, and if he does not get treatment, he may eventually develop convulsions and go into a coma. With medication the condition can be rapidly relieved and with a carefully controlled diet—a low protein diet—the dog can often be kept healthy and active for a long time. Generally, however, nephritis remains a potential danger, and in most cases the animal must be continued on a restricted diet for the rest of his life.

Another form of inflammatory kidney disease, called *pyelonephritis,* is often confused with the more common nephritis. But unlike nephritis, it affects only parts of the kidney. It is caused by one of several different types of bacteria. The chief difficulty is in identifying the specific bacteria involved, but once that has been done, the condition can be treated with very effective medications.

The failure of the kidneys to function adequately over a long period eventually results in the slow buildup of excessive amounts of uric acid in the blood. This condition, called *uremia,* is also fairly common in old dogs. It can be stubbornly persistent, and even to make a proper diagnosis often requires a number of tests and analyses. But if it is caught in time, the veterinarian can provide treatment to check its development and correct it.

The Urinary Bladder

. . . is perhaps the most common site of urinary difficulties with old dogs. The bladder is subject to infections of many kinds, and any excessive discharge from the vulva or penis should be given immediate attention. The infection may at first be the result of no more than a local infection which can easily be cleared up. But to let it go untreated is only to give the infection time to ascend from the bladder to the kidneys, where it may cause great difficulties.

Probably the most common of the bladder problems is an inflammation called *cystitis.* It is usually thought to begin with a bacterial infection, but there is some reason to believe that a virus of some sort may also be involved. It seems to be more prevalent among females than males, but both are susceptible. The first signs are that the dog seems to have some pain—perhaps a burning sensation—when he urinates. He is able to urinate only a little at a time after a long wait, and when he does he often whimpers in pain. Later there are signs of pus in the urine. The condition is treatable, but obviously it requires prompt attention.

Urinary calculi—bladder stones—are far more common than most owners realize. What causes them we still do not know. For some reason various kinds of salts in the urine sometimes precipitate out in the bladder and form accretions which—some authorities believe—begin by clustering around clumps of bacteria collected from infections. These stones—some visible by x-ray and some not, some smooth and rounded and some sharp and faceted—often continue to grow until they become the size of a Ping-Pong ball or larger. They are sometimes so large that they can be felt through the abdominal wall—if the dog is not obese—and owners are generally shocked and unbelieving when they are shown a fair specimen. Surprisingly, some dogs seem to be bothered very little even after the stones have grown quite large. Others very soon show signs of discomfort and pain. They often have difficulty in urinating, and sometimes there is bleeding and signs of an infection. Occasionally small stones will block the urethra—the tube leading from the bladder to the outside—and completely prevent the passage of urine. This is, of course, an acutely painful and dangerous condition which demands immediate attention. Surgery is the only solution for stones, and today the techniques are such that the danger is minimal and recovery is usually rapid.

Less frequently stones are formed in the kidneys. Usually they remain there, but now and then one may lodge in the ureter, the narrow tube which conducts the urine from the kidney to the bladder. People who have had a kidney stone will tell you that the pain is the most acute they have ever known—and presumably it is equally severe in dogs. Again, surgery is the only cure.

Urinary Incontinence

. . . compared to the painful kidney and bladder conditions we have been discussing, seems like a trifling problem. And it is—usually. But because owners are often unaware that it is a simple difficulty that can easily be corrected, it sometimes becomes a cruel and prolonged crisis.

Every year, it seems to me, I encounter half a dozen variations of the problem. A dejected client brings an old but still responsive dog to the office. "Doctor, here is old Penelope," he begins gravely. "We've decided that you'll have to put her to sleep. Oh, she looks good, I know. And she is good—in every way except one. When she sleeps she dribbles out water. It used to be only a little, but for the last year it has been a puddle every time. She sleeps at the foot of our bed. And even though we have a rubber sheet for her—well, the whole house smells, and we just can't stand it any longer. I'm sorry. I'm awful sorry."

The details vary, but the story is always the same. And only a person who has never felt an owner's heartbreak at the thought of losing a good old dog could smile at it.

It's a sad story, really, and a sad commentary on the failure of veterinarians to establish usable lines of communication with their clients.

Dribbling is usually a next-to-nothing problem. It is simply the result of a lack of a hormone, and generally it has been caused by an ovariohysterectomy which the dog had when she was a puppy. Occasionally—but much less frequently—an unspayed female will develop the same problem. In either case the treatment is quick, easy, and almost always effective. A telephone call is all it takes. Over the phone I can prescribe medication, the client can pick it up at any pharmacy and save himself months of distress and discomfort and the needless agony of deciding at last to give up a good old dog. All for a phone call.

But—there *is* a good side to the story. Can you imagine the owner's feelings when I tell him that Penelope's problem will have completely disappeared by the day after tomorrow?

The Reproductive System

. . . has its full share of ills, but they are fewer, of course, among old dogs than among those in the breeding age.

As a dog grows older his testicles normally shrink and become less firm. But in some cases an inflammation may cause one or both to become painfully enlarged, and in time the swelling may involve the scrotum as well. Unless the infection has been allowed to spread widely, medication is usually sufficient to clear up the condition. Drugs can be used to alleviate the pain until the treatment is effective.

Growths on or in one or both of the testicles are not uncommon in old dogs. Sometimes a growth in one will cause the other to atrophy. In such cases a dog will often lose his sex drive and sometimes he will acquire distinctly feminine characteristics. Surgery is generally necessary, but the removal of the affected testicle will often restore both the dog's masculinity and his potency.

Troubles with an enlarged prostate are even more common in old dogs. If they are untreated, the dog will in time have difficulty in passing stools and, still later, with urinating. Fortunately, however, the veterinarian will often discover the condition in the course of a routine examination before these overt symptoms appear. Though tumors do occasionally appear in the prostate, they are not common, and surgery is rarely necessary. Far more frequent are deep-seated infections which are, unfortunately, extremely resistant to medication and difficult to cure. Unless the dog is a valuable stud animal, veterinarians often recommend castration, which generally causes the prostate to shrink considerably, often within three or four weeks after the operation. But the condition must be treated, because an enlarged prostate causes a sensation like that of accumulated fecal material in the colon; the dog is likely to strain so hard to pass it that he will rupture himself. Castration will not change the dog's character, and in other important ways it may benefit him. I have no statistics to cite, but it has been my experience that castrated dogs generally live longer than their unaltered brethren.

And it might also be said here again that the same

is true—even more obviously and certainly true, I think —of the spayed female. Why the intact bitch has a shorter life than her spayed sister has still not definitely been determined, but there can hardly be any remaining doubt that she has. Even if birth-related deaths are ruled out entirely, I am convinced that the female who has had an ovariohysterectomy lives a year and a half to two years longer on the average than an unspayed animal. And two years is certainly a significant chunk of any dog's life.

In old female dogs the most common—and the most difficult—problem is an infection of the uterus called *pyometra.* It is a serious threat and one which very rapidly develops from nothing to a panic-button situation. One of the difficulties is that the early symptoms are so mild that they are easily overlooked, and the owner is seldom aware that the condition exists until it has reached a dangerous stage. At the beginning Penelope merely seems lackadaisical and listless. She often sleeps a great deal and usually she has little or no interest in food. These symptoms are hardly the warning signs one would expect in a developing crisis. But they may well be just that.

What happens in pyometra is that during a heat period the cervix is wide open and offers ready passage for infecting organisms to enter the uterus. At the end of the period the cervix closes tightly and the bacteria begin to proliferate at an extraordinary rate. The uterus, which is capable of expanding enough to hold a large litter of pups, begins to fill with pus. A few bacteria doubling and doubling again until they have become a few thousand cause little difficulty and few symptoms. But when cupfuls of pus collect and begin to double every few days, the uterus is soon filled to capacity. The body is saturated with toxins and the heart, the liver, and the kidneys may be so overburdened that the dog will suddenly become an emergency case. At this point in perhaps half the cases, the cervix is forced to dilate and the sticky, evil-smelling material seeps out, sometimes in pools. But that does not eliminate the infection. Usually there is no alternative to surgery, and only emergency treatment and intensive aftercare will save the dog.

Cysts and *tumors* sometimes appear in or around the ovaries. They are difficult to detect, and often a radiograph is necessary for diagnosis. Tumors are relatively rare, but cysts are somewhat more common. Fortunately, they may be present for years without creating any apparent difficulty, and even if they are known to exist, they can safely be ignored if they do not cause trouble. Those that do can usually be removed easily and safely by surgery.

In an old female the place where destructive tumors are most likely to appear is in the mammary area. These growths have been discussed in the section on cancer.

Diabetes

. . . *diabetes mellitus,* or sugar diabetes as it is commonly called, is often mistakenly thought to be a kidney-related problem because its diagnosis and control is associated with urinalysis. It is not. It is caused by an inadequate supply of the hormone insulin, which is necessary to keep the level of blood sugar within proper limits.

When the blood sugar rises beyond the acceptable level, some of it, together with an excessive amount of water, is eliminated through the kidneys. This increases the frequency and amount of urination and causes an excessive thirst to make up for the loss of water. If the condition is allowed to continue, there is a related increase in fat breakdown and that, in turn, creates a toxic condition throughout the body. The symptoms at this stage are labored breathing, general depression, vomiting, and eventually coma and death. In severe cases there may be a sweetish odor to the breath.

Fortunately, the symptoms are evident enough and disturbing enough so that the dog generally gets to the veterinarian before he goes into coma. It often happens that old Hector is brought in for an examination, not because the owner has recognized the early signs of diabetes, but because he has developed an eye problem. If it turns out that the dog's vision is being impaired by cataracts, the veterinarian will suspect that he is also diabetic because cataracts often occur in conjunction with the disease. The diagnosis can be confirmed, however, only by tests which measure the elevation of the blood sugar.

(Here, as elsewhere in this book, the masculine pronoun is used simply because it fits the manmade conventions of English grammar. The use of the masculine form in this case is not only regrettable. It is statistically wrong. For some reason as yet unknown, diabetes in dogs occurs almost five times as frequently in females as in males.)

With a diagnosis of diabetes, a blood sample is taken for analysis and an injection of insulin is given quickly to reduce the level of the blood sugar. Further tests are made frequently for at least the next twenty-four hours, and over the next few days injections are given as needed to regulate the condition. The dog is given measured quantities of food at regular intervals, and the amount of insulin is adjusted until the sugar in the blood is brought back to the desired level. After a few days, when the dog's condition has been firmly stabilized, he can be taken home. He is not *cured.* Nor will he ever be. But with conscientious care and careful supervision, there is no reason why he cannot live a near-normal life for many years.

Medically the treatment is not difficult, but as I have said elsewhere in this book, it is sometimes hard for an owner to accustom himself to the thought that jabbing a needle into his dog must thereafter become part of his daily schedule. But after he has reconciled himself to that necessity and has wielded the needle for a little while, giving the dog his insulin shot becomes a routine event which causes very little distress for either the one who gives or the one who receives.

It is unfortunate that there is still no effective substitute for the needle. A number of products which can be taken orally have been developed for the control of diabetes in people and in some cases, at least, they seem to work sufficiently well. Naturally, owners who have themselves used oral products or have heard of their use have been urgently demanding that they be prescribed for their diabetic dogs. I can only tell you that I have tried all of these products as they became available, and I must report that I have found that with dogs they are—in a word—worthless. I have decided that trying to use them is a waste of time—critically valuable time—which may well cost the dog's life.

The activities of a diabetic dog must forever be strictly regulated. His exercise has to be controlled. In a sudden burst of activity he will expend an unusual amount of energy, burn up sugar, and throw his system out of kilter. He will, therefore, have to become a leash dog. His diet will have to be strictly regulated with an established carbohydrate content, because as the carbohydrates vary, so does the blood sugar. He must get his shots and his food at regular intervals. And he has to be rigorously protected from the thoughtless kindness of his owner, the family, and family friends. Many a dog sails along in fine shape for months on a properly regulated food-insulin-exercise schedule—until the big cookout with all of its excitement and handouts. Until owners learn that for a diabetic dog there can be no free and easy weekends, veterinarians will continue to have a constant, depressing parade of Monday morning crises.

Once in a while a dog with a mild or arrested diabetic condition can get along well enough on a diet high in proteins and low in carbohydrates. If the veterinarian thinks that a restricted diet alone may be sufficient to control the sugar level, he will, of course, try it. Usually he will prescribe a very strictly controlled diet fed at regular hours twice a day. Diet sometimes works, but don't get your hopes too high. The odds are that in the end insulin injections will be necessary.

The routine care of a diabetic dog is demanding, and when you are first faced with it you may feel that it requires an unending series of tedious and distasteful chores. But in practice it becomes far less difficult than it seems in the telling. If you do have qualms and fears, you should discuss them frankly with your veterinarian. He has worked with people with the same problems many times before, and his experience with similar situations will undoubtedly be helpful.

There is another and quite different type of diabetes called *diabetes insipidus*. It involves the function of the hypothalamus, which is located at the base of the brain. It is not a sugar or insulin problem and is much less common than sugar diabetes. It is treated with injections of a hormone at intervals of twenty-four to seventy-two hours, depending upon the severity of the condition.

THE LIVER

. . . the largest and in many ways the busiest organ of the body is perhaps the least understood and least honored of all of them. (Except, of course, in parts of Europe, where it is still considered the king of organs and the source of most of the blessings and all of the ills of mankind.) In dogs, as in people, it does perform an enormous number of functions. By actual count, the liver, together with the gallbladder—which is a kind of subordinate and assistant—is involved in some two hundred separate and distinct processes. It produces bile, which is essential in the digestive process, takes sugar from the blood and stores it as glycogen, regulates clotting of the blood, converts waste products for elimination by the kidneys, creates antibodies for the protection of the system, synthesizes proteins, stores iron and copper salts, and—in the patter of the huckster—much, much more.

You would expect that in an old dog a host of difficulties would occur in an organ involved in so many functions of the body. And, in fact, a number do, but fewer and far less frequently than you would think. The liver is well protected from blows and external injuries by the rib cage, it is stubbornly resistant to toxins and poisons, and it has an overbuilt capacity that makes it possible for it to continue to function adequately even after it has been severely damaged by long abuse.

The most evident (and often the first) sign of a malfunctioning liver is *jaundice*—which, contrary to what most people think, is a *symptom* and not a disease. The bile which the liver produces is a yellowish substance, and when the presence of an excessive amount of it begins to discolor various tissues—the whites of the eyes, the skin, the gums—it is an indication that one of the many functions of the liver is out of kilter. It is a clear and urgent warning that your dog needs the attention of a veterinarian. There are too many possibilities for you to try guessing what is wrong.

Jaundice is not the only sign of a liver problem. Usually there is also a gradual decline in the dog's appetite, often enough to cause a loss of weight in time. The dog may vomit some, generally not violently but often frequently. He will be listless. In the later stages fluid will collect in his body, and often his abdomen will become distended. In many cases the veterinarian will be able to determine the specific causes of the symptoms only after he has the results of laboratory tests and blood analyses. And it is important that these be obtained promptly, for in some liver conditions early diagnosis is the difference between life and death.

In some old dogs degenerative changes occur in the liver. This is most likely to happen with those who have had severe bouts with diseases and infections which produced outpourings of toxins which (in the jargon) *insulted* the liver over prolonged periods. If the liver has been so damaged that its function is barely adequate under normal conditions, any sudden or excessive demand may stress it beyond its capacity. Fortunately, when that happens, the load can often be eased either by medication or by special diets.

Another condition, called *obstructive jaundice,* is not uncommon in old dogs. The bile produced by the liver is stored in the gallbladder, and from there it passes into the small intestine, where it aids in the digestion of fat, among other things. Anything which obstructs the bile duct—it could be an inflammation, stones, a tumor—may prevent the passage of sufficient bile and interfere with the digestive process. Nausea and vomiting are the usual early signs and they are caused not only by digestive difficulties but also by the toxic effects of the bile backing up in the liver. The condition can be treated in a number of ways, depending both on its cause and severity. But it is serious, and the dog must have prompt attention.

By no means all conditions which cause jaundice or appear to be liver ailments are caused by the malfunctioning of the liver itself. That organ is complexly related to many functions of the body and can be severely and immediately affected by failures anywhere in the system. To take only one example: a decrease in blood pressure can cause acute and critical changes in the function of the liver. The liver problem, then, might be the result of cardiac insufficiency. Or it might be brought on by the increasing effects of arteriosclerosis. Or—less obviously but, unhappily, with increasing frequency of late—it could be the result of a heavy infestation of heartworms. And the list might go on. . . .

The symptoms of liver disorders are not difficult to recognize. Any owner ought to be able to see that something is wrong with his dog. But they *are* difficult to interpret. And that means that the diagnosis will have to be made by a veterinarian and not by the owner.

Hepatitis

. . . *infectious canine hepatitis* is a viral disease which causes an inflammation of the liver—and for that reason it is mentioned here. An effective vaccine is available today, and all puppies should be properly inoculated against the disease. It has been my experience that it occurs mainly, almost exclusively, in young dogs. You will be happy to know that since I have never heard of a case of hepatitis in a dog over eleven years old, I think there is no need for you to be concerned about it.

Leptospirosis

. . . is a bacterial disease which affects both the kidneys and the liver. There are, in fact, several different types of the disease, but one of the diagnostic symptoms common to all serious cases of any of them is the jaundiced appearance characteristic of liver ailments. Though leptospirosis is usually a mild disease and seldom actually causes death, in some areas it is a threat, particularly to show dogs, who come in frequent contact with others who may be carrying the disease—which is, by the way, communicable to people. There is, fortunately, an effective preventive inoculation. Its chief drawback is that to be fully protected the dog must be inoculated every six months.

The Digestive System

. . . from lips to anus, is a long passageway which, though it is within the body, is open to the exterior and thus is properly considered part of the *outside* of the body, a continuation of the skin. It is, we say, a single system, but it is composed of a great many parts, each with a specialized function in the complicated process of converting food into substances to build, nourish, sustain, and repair the body. Its functions are both mechanical and chemical. It includes the mouth, lips, teeth, esophagus, stomach, and the small and large intestines. From beginning to end it is some five or six times as long as the dog himself.

The list of possible ills, ailments, and disruptions is as long as the digestive system itself. Many of them are rare and anomalous conditions that can and do occur unreasonably and unpredictably, but they are problems to test the skills and addle the minds of veterinarians. Happily old dogs do develop certain immunities and resistances. And even though the aging process does to some extent affect the digestive system adversely, in many ways it actually becomes more efficient as the dog grows older. What we are concerned with here are the common, the probable, the usual difficulties your old dog may encounter. There are enough of them, surely, but not so many that you will become unhinged and unhappy with the outlook for the future.

The dog's mouth and teeth should get a good deal more attention than they usually do. Any troubles that develop in that area can easily be seen by the owner, and you would think that he would be quick to report them as soon as they appear. Not so. Instead, many—indeed, most—owners neglect them scandalously. A foul breath is unmistakable—and an unmistakable sign that something is wrong. Yet I have many clients who delay bringing in their dogs until the animal's breath is a stench in the examining room, and I wonder how the owner could have lived with the odor in his house. Sometimes the dog's teeth are obviously loose or broken, or they are buried in tartar and the gums are bleeding. Sometimes he is suffering with a protruding growth in his mouth or on his lips that clearly must have troubled him for weeks or months. No owner can fail to see obvious problems of this sort. And if he is at all observant he should also see and respond to less urgent signs of developing problems. If a dog drools a great deal after drinking, or if he seems to be working his tongue in his mouth constantly, or if he has chronic and persistent difficulty in swallowing, he needs to be examined by a veterinarian promptly.

His *teeth* are often an old dog's strongest point, and I have often seen ancient animals whose teeth and gums are in magnificent shape. And even though a dog may have an isolated tooth problem or two, his teeth generally remain in reasonably good condition until the aging process is well along. There are, as always, exceptions. In my opinion, bad teeth in younger dogs are usually the result of genetic factors. Some strains of Yorkshire Terriers, for example, commonly lose as many as half their teeth by the time they are four or five years old—and I know of nothing that can be done to prevent that. Neglect can and will ruin the best mouth in the world, of course. But a dog that starts with a good set of teeth and the right genes is not likely to have many dental problems. Cavities in dogs' teeth are rare—so rare that I collect teeth with caries as specimens. Candy and sweets have no harmful effects that I have been able to discover. Nor does the consistency of a dog's diet seem to make any difference in the condition of his teeth. Many old dogs have beautiful teeth and healthy gums after a lifetime of eating nothing but soft, mushy food.

Tartar is the main troublemaker. On some dogs' teeth it builds up to such thickness that it forces the gums to recede severely. Pockets of pus and infection first form between the tartar and the gums and then work back under the gums to the roots and cause the teeth to loosen. Prevention is the remedy. By occasionally using a damp wad of cotton dipped in ordinary powdered pumice (available at any drugstore) the owner himself can remove the soft tartar before it is converted to the stony stuff that does the damage. But after it has accumulated for years and hardened, removing it is a job for the veterinarian. And it is not an easy or pleasant one.

When a tooth becomes infected, it should be removed

promptly. It won't get better, and one bad tooth generally infects those on either side of it. In addition, there is good evidence that the bacteria is carried to other parts of the body where it often causes serious problems. When the tooth is extracted, the infection usually clears up quickly and the old dog may well go along for years without any further dental problems.

In old dogs a swelling sometimes appears under one eye, and if it isn't treated in time, it will often rupture and drain. More often than not the lesion is caused by an infection in the root of a tooth and after the tooth is extracted the swelling will disappear. Occasionally when an upper canine tooth is removed an opening from the root of the tooth to the nasal cavity remains. Until the gums heal, food sometimes works up through the opening and causes the dog to sneeze. This debris should be removed, for if it is not, it may start a nasal infection.

Some people think that giving old Hector bones to chew helps to keep his teeth healthy. And it is true that for him gnawing at a bone can be a pleasurable (if not very effective) way of removing some of the tartar. But there are disadvantages to be considered, too. If the dog wallows the bone around where there have been feces and worm eggs, he is greatly increasing his chances of infestation. There is also the danger that he will swallow a sharp splinter which can seriously injure him. If you do give the dog a bone, at least make sure that it is a hard marrowbone or a knucklebone—and to be safe, take it away from him before he works it down to the splintering stage. If you can't bring yourself to deprive him of those final moments of pleasure, bake the bone in the oven for four or five hours before you give it to him. That will make it virtually indestructible.

Some old dogs never seem to outgrow the habit (or need) to chew things that they shouldn't—sticks, stones, pipes, bones of exactly the wrong size or shape—and occasionally they contrive to get a piece of one of these things wedged between their upper back molars. When that happens, they will drool, rub their heads along the ground, scratch and paw at their faces in a vain effort to get rid of the obstruction. If your dog suddenly engages in antics of this sort, open his mouth and look for his problem. If you can't work the obstruction loose with your fingers, try using a pair of long-nosed pliers. If that doesn't work, take the dog to the veterinarian before he (the dog, that is) becomes frantic.

Even if your dog is genetically blessed and seems to have sound teeth, when he gets old it is prudent to have the veterinarian examine them from time to time—as he routinely will if the dog is taken in for an annual checkup. But it is time to take him in whenever there are signs of any tooth problem, and if it turns out to be at all serious, the dog will probably be put on a six-month examination schedule.

Bad breath is not always caused by bad teeth. Often the cause is a rather common infection in the fold of the lower lip, usually in the area opposite the canine teeth. If you run your finger along the fold, you will find that it comes away with a very foul odor. The condition is not serious, but it is annoying for the dog and it must certainly be unpleasant for the owner. There is no need for either to suffer. The infection can be cleared up quickly with a little medication.

Tumors of the gums are not uncommon. And—presumably for genetic reasons, again—they occur more frequently in some breeds than in others. Boxers especially are prone to such tumors as they grow older. These growths are called *epulis*. Though they are generally nuisances rather than dangers, they sometimes grow large enough to make it difficult for the dog to chew comfortably. In such cases they should be removed.

Tumors also appear in other parts of the mouth, and there is recent evidence that they are becoming increasingly common. A report from the University of Pennsylvania, for example, indicates that in dogs the mouth and throat are the most frequent sites of growths today. It has also been shown that city dogs have a much higher incidence of mouth tumors than farm dogs, and it is thought that the difference may be due to environmental factors, probably pollutants carried in the air. Whatever the reason, the increase is a cause for real alarm, for both dogs and people are exposed to the same hazards and often suffer the same consequences.

Tumors of the mouth and lips may be either malignant or benign. The latter, often *polyps* and *papillomas,* are not dangerous and can be easily and permanently removed. But others cannot be so readily identified and often tissue must be submitted to a pathologist for analysis. The mouth is an area where pigmented tumors frequently appear, and they are among the most devastating growths a dog can get. They are always difficult, and only early diagnosis and radical surgery, when it is possible, will save the dog's life.

Dogs are susceptible to a number of conditions which affect the throat and esophagus, but in my practice I find that such ills are not very common in old dogs. *Pharyngitis* and *laryngitis* seldom occur, and *tonsillitis* is also fairly infrequent largely, I suppose, because the dogs have built up substantial immunity over the years. They do get an occasional local infection in this area, but generally it can be treated and eliminated handily.

And always, of course, there is the danger of punctures, cuts and scrapes in the throat if the dog attempts to swallow some impossible object. Injuries of this sort are generally less likely to occur as the dog grows older. But it is still worth a sentence to remind you that some dogs are never totally immune to strange, attractive objects. Never a year passes without my seeing at least a few painfully injured dogs—oldsters as well as puppies—who were simply unable to resist sampling such things as lures and fishhooks dangling within their reach.

The most serious of the old dog's digestive problems occur either in the *stomach* or in the small or large *intestines,* and to understand them you should know a little about how his digestive system works. In a dog's stomach food is subjected to acids almost twice as strong as those in the human stomach—so strong that the toughest muscle meats and even bones can be broken down for further digestion. Some digestive enzymes are added here and some later when the acidified food passes into the small intestines. There the bile from the liver and the pancreatic juices are introduced. These change the mixture from acid to alkaline and promote a breakdown of the food so that the nutritional elements can be absorbed into the blood. As the foodstuff leaves the small intestine, it is still quite fluid, but during the passage through the large intestine it is gradually dehydrated until it passes out of the body as a relatively firm mass.

In a process that long and complicated there can be failures anywhere along the line. A physical obstruction or a stoppage, either partial or complete and at any point, can create a problem. The block could be caused by a tumor, or by the growth of scar tissue, or by a mass of indigestible material of any sort, or by a twist or snarl in the intestines—anything which prevents the programmed movement of the food material. The failure of the body to produce sufficient enzymes or the failure to deliver them in the proper quantities to the proper place at the proper time can throw the system out of gear. Too much or too little acid can upset the process. Poisons, toxic substances and infections can create havoc. If peristalsis, the motion of the digestive tract which carries the food along, slows down or stops or—as it sometimes does—reverses, the process is brought to a halt.

In a system so complex it is often difficult to determine the immediate and specific cause of any malfunction. And indeed, it often happens that there is no single cause for a condition but rather a number of interrelated factors that are involved. A whole spectrum of symptoms is often present, but the most common and most evident signs of a problem somewhere in the digestive system are nausea and vomiting, diarrhea and constipation—or some combination of all three.

These symptoms in themselves are seldom sufficient to pinpoint the difficulty, but they are sometimes at least helpful in pointing the direction the investigation must take. Vomiting is the most common and least informative of the signs. It is associated with so many problems that it points in all directions at once. As a symptom, diarrhea is a little better. It can generally be assumed that diarrhea *without* nausea and vomiting is indicative of a problem centered in the large intestine. Diarrhea *with* vomiting suggests that the difficulty is likely to be located in the stomach or the small intestine. These problems, unlike those in the large intestine, generally cause considerable pain and distress, and on the whole they tend to be more serious than those of the large intestine. Constipation is not only a symptom of a multitude of possible difficulties, but a problem in itself. More about that later.

But at best these are no more than first clues. Consider the possibilities in one simple, common case. An old dog develops loose stools, and they persist for some time. But he doesn't vomit and he shows no loss of appetite. As a starter, the veterinarian may assume that the problem is in the lower bowel. But many conditions can cause an outpouring of fluid and produce a loose stool—the diet itself or even a change in one of the components of a diet; the presence of some toxic substance; an inflammation of some sort; an infection; even a local irritation. Some people think that when a dog drinks an excessive amount of water, it runs right down the intestinal tract and out through the bowel and kidneys. It doesn't, of course. The water that is drunk is absorbed into the system from the stomach, and if too much water appears in the bowel movement, it is because it has been returned through the intestinal wall.

And so the veterinarian must go on to discover which of many possible conditions has caused *that* to happen, and before he finds the answer—and the means to correct it—he may well have to perform a whole series of tests.

Or, take another case—one in which the old dog *is* vomiting. It is quite possible that he has incautiously licked up something that is sufficiently irritating to cause the stomach to empty itself. But if there is a yellowish-green substance in the material that has been regurgitated, that indicates that some of the bile in the small intestine has returned to the stomach either before or during the vomiting. Too much bile—or too little, for that matter—can create a digestive disturbance. But so can an excess or deficiency of pancreatic juices. Both produce much the same symptoms—about the same kind and amount of vomiting and the same depression. But with pancreatitis there is severe pain, and when the bile backs up there is usually much less. Usually—but, of course, not always. And so, once again, the veterinarian has to make further examinations and get further tests before he can make a diagnosis.

And while he is about them, he must also remember that a tumor of the stomach can make a dog a chronic vomiter. Or that there may be an obstruction in the intestine. Or that the valve at the exit of the stomach may not be functioning properly.

It is not easy to discover the cause of a digestive problem. For anybody. And for the layman it is next to impossible.

That is not to say that all problems connected with the digestive system are skull-busting puzzles. Many of them aren't. Many an old dog has been made violently sick by taking a casual lick of some toxic substance—and returned to the bloom of health by a simple stomach coater. And it often turns out that the food that an old dog has been eating for years has simply become too difficult for his aging system to handle. In that case a simple change of diet may make him as fit as he ever was. Or he may need a specialized diet to fit the changing flow of acids and enzymes, a diet long on one element and short on another.

Once in a while, when I have been baffled by the problems of an old dog whose system has been laboring along with some undefinable difficulty, I have prescribed a diet which is intended simply to normalize stools that are either too loose or too firm. It is made up of equal parts by volume of stewed tomatoes, cooked hamburger, and rice. I know that it sounds like a fad diet. And I warn owners that since it is lacking in all sorts of essential elements, it can be used for only a limited time. But it works. I admit that I don't know exactly how or why. But in many cases it does work. I have seen many a dilapidated old dog's system right itself after a few days of this diet—and stay right.

One cause of simple digestive problems that keeps popping up—and one that few owners ever think of—is that an old dog may suddenly, and for no apparent reason, become sensitive to one or another of the ingredients in the commercial food that he has been eating for years. The producers of dog foods do change their formulas from time to time, and though they usually add enough coloring matter to make the new product look to you just like the one you have always been getting, your dog may discover the difference. Or the manufacturer may merely shift the proportions a bit. If your dog has a little difficulty in digesting fish meal and the producer decides to increase the fish meal by 20 percent to jack up the protein content of the food, you may have a vomiting problem on your hands. You can easily solve the problem by shifting to a food in which the protein is less fishy, but I have known many cases in which it took months to discover that the solution was so simple.

Constipation is a common problem among old dogs,

and one that is frequently made uncommonly difficult because owners either fail to recognize it or to do anything about it until it has become a threat to the dog's health.

It is difficult to see how an owner can fail to notice the symptoms. Usually the dog assumes the position for defecating and remains that way for a long time without results, often with much straining. If he is at last able to pass a hard, cementlike stool, it is sometimes so painful that he will whimper and cry. If the condition becomes chronic, he will lose his appetite and his abdomen will become distended. He will often become depressed and apprehensive. His breath will be foul. In extreme cases a dog may even digest his food and later regurgitate the fecal material. The bowel can be totally blocked. I have known scandalously neglected dogs who have somehow managed to survive for weeks without once being able to evacuate.

Once again, prevention is the remedy. There are dozens of reasons for an old dog becoming constipated, and almost all of them can easily be avoided or prevented. Here is a short list—with a few comments that should be unnecessary.

Hector is generally allowed to put on weight as he grows older. The older he gets, the less active he becomes; and the heavier he is, the less exercise he gets. An overweight dog is always more likely to become constipated than a dog that is kept in good shape.

If a dog isn't given as much water as he needs, the food descending to the lower bowel may become so dehydrated that it causes constipation. Solution: more water.

Some foods are by their nature constipating—bones, muscle meat, dog biscuits. They should be fed sparingly or not at all to a dog that has a tendency to be constipated.

A shocking number of old dogs with long hair around the anal area develop something that should be called obstructive constipation. It is caused, unbelievably, by the owner's allowing dried feces to collect in the hair until it interferes with the passage of stools. Scissors will cure the condition.

Too much medication—or the owner's willingness to medicate rather than to eliminate the cause of the condition permanently by improving the dog's diet—often causes constipation or exacerbates it. Some drugs which first act as a physic actually cause constipation later. And medicines used to prevent loose stools sometimes do their work only too well. No dog should be constantly or whimsically dosed with drugs to regulate his bowel movements.

There are other causes of constipation which the owner can't prevent or control, but they are far less common than those listed above. In an old dog an enlarged prostate, whether due to a tumor or an infection, can become an obstruction to the lower bowel that makes defecation painful or even impossible. In such cases, the constipation can be permanently eliminated only by the proper treatment of the prostate, which is discussed elsewhere. The failure of the gallbladder to provide sufficient bile may also lead to constipation. The bile deficiency can be treated. Posterior paralysis or an injury to the nerves activating the lower bowel may reduce the activity of the bowel so that fecal material becomes impacted, or leave the bowel entirely inactive. These are, of course, disastrous situations, always difficult and often impossible to treat.

Constipation of the usual kind—the sort that is the result of neglect—simply shouldn't be allowed to happen. When it does, the basic causes (usually dietary) should be eliminated and the existing constipation remedied as gently and as naturally as possible. A good-sized bowl of skimmed milk is an excellent laxative for most dogs. It is well known, too, that liver produces a loose stool. And, if the dog's system easily tolerates fat, he can be fed an increased amount which will enter the bowel and lubricate the stool so that it can be passed more easily.

When the problem has been allowed to become more

serious, a limited amount of medication may be necessary. Mineral oil given over a period of a few days slowly softens and lubricates the fecal material so that it can be passed. Sometimes glycerin suppositories or Fleet enemas are helpful, but they should not be used often or regularly. If the situation has become an emergency, the veterinarian may have to give the dog enemas, using literally gallons of water to break down the accumulation and wash it away. Occasionally he may have to prescribe drugs as stool softeners. And now and then, when constipation has been permitted to exist for an unconscionable time and dehydration is present, he may even be forced to administer intravenous fluids, sometimes with B-complex, in a desperate effort to save the old dog's life.

The usual cause of constipation, I repeat, is neglect. Proper diet is the surest preventive and the soundest cure.

The anal glands, sometimes called "scent glands," are located on either side of and a little below the anus. They secrete a liquid which is normally discharged through ducts into the anus. But sometimes—even in young dogs, but more often in older animals—the secretion collects in the glands and becomes a thick, gummy mass with an offensive odor. The impacted material often makes the dog uncomfortable and causes him to drag his rear along the ground or to lick himself excessively. By exerting a little pressure on the gland the veterinarian can express the contents and relieve the dog. It is not difficult, but there is a bit of a trick to doing it quickly and easily. If the problem is a recurrent one with your dog, your veterinarian can show you how you can clear the glands at home.

The Skin

. . . is an organ, just as the liver and the heart and the lungs are. It includes not only the visible, external part which encases the body, but also the mucous membranes which line body cavities such as the nose, mouth, eyes, and digestive tract. But usually the skin is thought of only as the external covering which holds the dog together and separates him from the world. And it is that part of the skin we are concerned with here. It is worth remembering, however, that the skin has many functions other than the obvious one of keeping the parts of the dog assembled in good order.

The dog's skin has been likened to a barometer which by its ills and changes reflects the general condition of the animal. And in some cases and to some degree that it true. But not always and not entirely. If some skin conditions are related to internal problems, there are many that are not. On the basis of the hard facts available today, we can only say that there are a multitude of factors that may—or may not—be involved in many skin conditions. Which is the long way of saying that we don't know.

In the maze of possible causes, veterinarians have found that diet is at least peripherally involved in a great many skin problems. It is generally impossible to establish a direct and specific connection. But this much can certainly be said: With any dog—and particularly with an old dog—an inadequate or improper diet adversely affects the condition of the skin and thus makes it more vulnerable to attack; and a good, well-balanced diet is always helpful in the treatment of any of the common skin problems.

It is especially important that an old dog be given a diet that is rich in high-quality protein that is readily available, includes as much fat as the dog can easily tolerate, and is amply supplied with the vitamins and trace minerals necessary for good health. It is a continual problem for the owner to provide the proper balance if the dog is fed largely on leftovers, and the table-scrap diet is almost always lacking in one essential or another. Many of the commercial foods now on the market—the dry foods and the semimoist foods, at least—do provide all of the known essentials. That being true, it seems to me both safer and easier to use a commercial food than to spend money on hit-and-miss supplements that are often useless if not downright injurious.

But providing the proper food is not the answer to all problems. A balanced diet is useless if the dog's system is unable to utilize the available nutriments. Digestive problems anywhere along the line can cancel out the benefits and set up conditions for the development of many kinds of skin disorders. An underactive thyroid gland is sometimes a contributing factor. A relatively slight malfunction in either the kidneys or the liver can create skin problems. An erratic or insufficient supply of bile or pancreatic juices which creates digestive problems can indirectly cause a skin ailment. Many such possibilities must be considered in the search for the elusive cause-cure solution to skin disorders.

An imbalance of hormones produced in the body can also be involved. This is especially true of old dogs in whom a natural change is already taking place. For example, in an old dog it is not uncommon for an insignificant-looking tumor in one testicle to so disturb the hormone balance that he will take on distinct female characteristics including a noticeable growth of the mammary glands. More surprising, he may also develop mammary tumors characteristic of the female as well as other unusual skin disorders. All of these disappear with the removal of the tumor and the testicle.

Finding the cause of a skin disorder, it is clear, is often the most difficult part of the problem. Once that has been determined, the outlook is much improved. Diet can be corrected, digestive problems can be eliminated, hormones can be supplied, and the skin condition itself will often disappear or readily yield to treatment. But the search—the search is often discouragingly long and frustrating.

But even when we don't fully understand what causes a skin condition—or even exactly what it is—we can often do something to relieve the distress and discomfort which it causes. And sometimes we can eliminate it altogether. Let me give you an example.

For years veterinarians have been contending as best they can with a skin rash which some dogs develop annually, usually in midsummer or early fall. Dogs often begin to get the attacks when they are young and generally the itch becomes worse each year until by the time the dogs are old it has become an annual misery. It is called *eczema* or *summer eczema* and sometimes just "summer itch" or "summer fungus" or "grass fungus"—a host of names, indicating I think, that nobody yet understands what it is or what causes it.

But whatever it is, for the dog it is an excruciating affliction. It usually begins on the back near the tail. In a day or so it spreads to the base of the tail itself, along the rear of the back legs and further up on the back. And sometimes it extends over the abdomen and keeps on spreading until it covers most of the animal's skin. The dog becomes frantic. He pulls out wads of hair and chews up and down his front legs as though he were eating corn on the cob. But that doesn't mean that only his front legs itch. He attacks them—sometimes until they bleed—simply out of frustration because he itches all over.

Something has to be done for a dog in such misery, and veterinarians have tried dozens of ways to make him at least a little more comfortable. Oral antibiotics and frequent medicated baths sometimes provide a measure of relief. If the dog continues in a frenzy of scratching and biting himself, the veterinarian may (pretty much out of desperation) resort to the use of steroids. They seem to help, but they cannot be given for long because of their undesirable side effects.

Owners and veterinarians are often so distressed by the dog's frantic scratching that they are willing to try almost anything that will provide even temporary relief. Once, when I had to tell a weary and discouraged client that he could not expect any real improvement in the dog's condition until after the first frost, he unexpectedly brightened up. He was a turkey farmer and he asked if I thought it would be all right if he took the dog with him into the walk-in freezer where he worked for an hour or so twice a week packing birds for freezing. Considering the condition of the old dog's lacerated skin, I thought that it could certainly do him no harm and might conceivably bring him some relief. A couple of weeks later the owner reported that the itching had completely stopped after the dog's first session in the cold and that he proposed to keep the dog in the freezer for half an hour twice a week until the cold weather set in.

That was hardly a workable solution for the general problem. Most owners aren't turkey farmers. I'm not sure that the health department would approve of the treatment. And it would be a bit outlandish to prescribe a walk-in freezer for the usual case of eczema.

But the fact that even a brief chilling of the dog's skin was enough to check the eczema for the season did lead to further thoughts. Dogs sweat very little. But it did seem at least possible that a spell of hot, humid weather might somehow trigger a change in the dog's skin which caused it to become more moist than usual—and perhaps to secrete some material that was irritating to the skin. If that was true, I thought, then anything that would keep down the moisture might prevent the miserable summer itch.

The following season when a dog with a long history of eczema was brought in, I asked and was given permission to try what I explained would probably be a hopeless—but certainly harmless—experiment. I sprayed the dog with an ordinary drugstore brand of antiperspirant. It seemed to help. I bought and tried several other standard varieties available in my neighborhood. Many of them gave the dogs some relief almost immediately. A powdered aerosol spray used daily for two or three days and then once every three days relieved the symptoms totally in many cases. I have since urged scores of owners to try it on their dogs and generally they have found that it worked as well as it did on the animals I used it on. And when it has failed, I suspect that it was used improperly or for conditions mistakenly thought to be eczema.

Mange, a skin disease caused by burrowing microscopic mites, is sometimes—particularly in its early stages—mistaken for other problems. There are two main types of mange and, aside from the fact that they affect the skin and cause intense itching, neither of them is related in any way to eczema. Both cause intense and persistent discomfort and both should be treated without delay when they appear.

Sarcoptic mange, though it is far more common in young dogs, does occur with some frequency in older ones. It appears in small spots which spread outward to become bald patches that the dog rakes and scratches incessantly. The mites (from which it takes its name) burrow deeply into the skin so that it is often difficult to collect enough of them for identification under the microscope. But once the diagnosis has been made, the treatment is simple. It should be prompt and thorough, for the disease can be transmitted from dogs to people and from people to people.

Demodectic mange, or red mange, was once such a persistent and unyielding affliction that veterinarians sometimes resorted to surgery in an effort to prevent it from becoming a creeping torment to the dog. Today it is not common as a disease among old dogs, although it is not unusual for a dog to carry mites without showing any obvious signs. Only rarely—very rarely, in my experience—is the disease transmitted to people. Most cases respond well to treatment with the medications now available. The chief problem is that the first symptoms are often so mild that the diagnosis is late and it sometimes takes considerable time to discover all of the affected spots and prevent the mites from attacking new areas.

Ringworm is a fungus infection. It is relatively rare but by no means unknown in older dogs. It usually starts as a small itchy spot that grows outward for a time—but not always with the neat geometry the name implies—and then appears in similar patches elsewhere on the body. It is militantly contagious and it can easily be picked up and exchanged among almost all of the members of the household—cats and children, pups, parents, and playmates. It can be eliminated with diligence and a good fungicide, but it should always be treated vigorously and soon.

Seborrhea is a functional disease in which the oil glands of the skin produce excessive secretions which coat the skin and hair with a waxlike substance that has a peculiarly pungent and disagreeable odor. What causes these glands to become overactive is not known, but the condition seems to be most common in older dogs. Seborrhea is a troublesome disease which can be controlled but not cured. Until we know more about the condition, medicated baths on a regular basis will have to serve as the most effective treatment.

There are many less serious skin and coat conditions that occasionally become nuisance problems with old dogs. The loss of hair, for example. Thinning hair is a normal sign of aging, but now and then it approaches *alopecia* which, less elegantly, is called baldness. If it is hereditary—and it may be—you will simply have to learn to love a balding dog. But sometimes it is a disease symptom (it might be diabetes) or a hormone imbalance (tumors associated with or affecting glands) and these conditions can often be corrected.

Dandruff—which does occur in some dogs, often only seasonally—may reflect a generally poor skin condition which can usually be improved. Often it is nothing more than the natural flaking of the outer skin—a cosmetic problem for which the best treatment is regular, vigorous brushing.

Psoriasis, a thickening and coarsening of the skin in local areas that is often called "elephant skin" by owners, is not uncommon in old dogs. Its cause is not known—it is different from the callouses which old dogs sometimes develop on elbows and other points of wear—but it can be treated with medications intended to help keep the skin pliable.

Sore spots and inflammation caused by stiff collars and heavy harness shouldn't happen at all. But when they do, they should be treated. Often they *don't* get well. They get infected.

Owners often ask if it is possible for a dog to get a *contact dermatitis* such as poison ivy. I think not. One summer and fall some years ago I conducted a less-than-definitive experiment. Using rubber gloves, I vigorously rubbed poison ivy leaves on the lower abdomens of ten Beagles twice a week for a couple of months. Not one dog developed the slightest blemish. But I did. I developed the worst case of poison ivy I have ever had. Dogs don't get poison ivy. But I should remind you that a dog running through a patch of poison ivy carries the stuff with him on his coat, and if you are susceptible, *you* can get it when you pet him.

A *flea collar* will occasionally cause a serious, stubborn inflammatory reaction in the skin of the dog's neck. The reaction, which is a true contact dermatitis, can be more than a mere disturbing nuisance. There have been cases in which old dogs in a weakened or debilitated condition have died from the effects. The inflammation generally is caused by an excessive amount of chemical in the collar. The problem can usually be avoided by removing the collar from the envelope in which it is sold and exposing it to the air for at least twelve hours before it is put on the dog. It is wise to look at the dog's neck a week after the collar is put on. If there is no sign of a reaction by that time, you can assume that the collar is safe.

Allergies

. . . in dogs are not, in my opinion, as common as they are sometimes thought to be, and there is still much doubt, dispute, and contention about many reactions that have rather casually been classified as allergic. However, there can now be little doubt that some dogs do indeed have a true allergic reaction to certain substances—most commonly, in my experience, to horsemeat and eggs among food items, and to such external substances as pollen, house dust, wool, and perhaps even some of the synthetic fibers. I have wrestled with enough cases in these areas to erase any lingering skepticism.

The problem with allergies is that there are hundreds of things in and around a dog which *could* cause his reaction, and to discover which of them is actually responsible can be a long and discouraging business. One rule of thumb approach to the problem—as unreliable as most rules are—is that if the condition (a loss of hair, for example) is general and symmetrical and is essentially identical on both sides of the dog's body, the cause is likely to be internal, probably dietary. But if the symptoms are *not* symmetrical and do not appear on both sides, the chances are that the cause is some external, environmental factor.

There are two ways to discover what is causing an allergy, and neither of them is easy. If the causative factor is thought to be something in the dog's diet, the usual method is to try to find out what it is by a process of elimination. The diet is first reduced to a single type of food. For example, the dog may be fed nothing but hamburger for a week. If, toward the end of that period, his condition has definitely improved, it can safely be assumed that the cause *is* some item in his diet, and that it is not hamburger. Thereafter a single ingredient is added to his food each week. As long as the dog has no reaction, you will know that none of the items he is eating is involved in his problem. But when you do at last add the substance to which he is allergic—it may be milk or fish or even one of the minor ingredients of a commercial food—the familiar symptoms will appear almost immediately.

The elimination process is a logical way to go about the search for the offending substance. And with a little bit of luck, it sometimes works remarkably well. But it is tediously time-consuming at best, and not infrequently it ends inconclusively or even with the discovery of further difficulties. Some dogs, for instance, have been found to be allergic to virtually all animal protein. And when that happens, the veterinarian has the problem of devising an adequate diet which includes only vegetable protein—and then persuading the dog that the doctor knows best.

Allergies caused by external factors are even more difficult to track down because the environment can't conveniently be reduced to a single element to which others can be added one by one. With environmental allergies the only practical way to determine the cause is by skin testing—a diagnostic method that few veterinarians are prepared to undertake. Investigations of this sort can best be handled at veterinary schools where proper facilities are available.

Not long ago I had a patient with a puzzling skin condition which I had treated with minimal success for nearly a year. When his owner told me that he planned to vacation high above Cayuga's waters, I suggested that he take the dog for skin tests at the veterinary school at Cornell. He did and they did—and after a few dozen tests it was discovered that the dog was allergic to kapok, of all things. He was desensitized by injections and now lives happily with kapok all around.

More often the offending substance is discovered only by happy accident. I remember one old dog who during a long life from time to time developed an excruciating itch. I treated him many times, and though lotions somewhat eased his discomfort on and off—mostly off—I was unhappy with the uncertain and unpredictable results. Both the owner and I had dismissed the possibility of an allergy because of the random and intermittent occurrence of the signs, but I had been unable to establish any other plausible diagnosis.

One summer the dog's owner rented a vacation cottage on a lake. Since it seemed possible that life in the wild—splashing in the lake and plowing through thickets and swamps—would trigger the itch, I supplied the owner with a goodly stock of lotions and pills. But instead of getting worse, the city dog's signs disappeared within a day after he got to the country. The medication was discontinued and the itch went away and stayed away—until the owner made a one-day visit to the city to replenish the camp supplies. He took the dog with him, and they had hardly driven five minutes from the lake until the dog was again frantic with the itch, biting and scratching and pulling his hair. But when he got back to the cottage in the evening, the dog began to recover immediately.

A week later master and dog drove to a nearby town, and again within minutes the symptoms reappeared with the same severity. But still, on day-long hikes miles from the camp the dog was untroubled. At last it occurred to us that it was the car that was causing his trouble. Not the car itself, it turned out, and not the motion—but the wool blanket that was used to protect the upholstery. The cottage was furnished in spare summer style—grass rugs, cotton bedding, wicker furniture, and no wool at all. In the house in the city the floor coverings were of synthetic materials, but there were woolen blankets and woolen upholstery and woolen clothing—enough to trouble the dog intermittently, but apparently not enough to produce the frenzy that direct contact with the car blanket had induced.

It is generally not feasible to pluck up a dog bodily

and drop him into an entirely new environment. But it is often possible to make changes in his routine that yield clues about the substances that may be causing allergic reactions. Many of them are thought to act primarily through the respiratory system and sometimes only when the substance is inhaled continuously for hours. Changing the place where the dog sleeps can cause a dramatic improvement. It may help if you merely move his bed from the basement to the garage. Or if you give him an entirely new kind of bedding material. Or let him sleep on the vinyl floor in the kitchen. Or discourage him from taking long afternoon snoozes on the woolen rug in the living room. Making such changes is admittedly a hit-or-miss approach, but it is possible that you will luck out and find the cause of the trouble. But failing that, you will have to go the skin-test route if the dog's difficulties become acute.

Testing can be a long and expensive way to discover what is causing an allergy. But with perseverance and patience it usually works, and in most cases the cause can either be eliminated or the dog desensitized. The worst that can happen is to discover that the dog is sensitive to himself. That is not a joke. It has been found that in rare cases a dog can become sensitive to a part of his own anatomy and reject it. If the condition is discovered early (as it seldom is, of course) and treated vigorously, it may be possible to save the dog. But in most cases, unfortunately, the situation is hopeless.

It seems unkind to add to your worries, but I should also remind you that some dogs have an allergic reaction to insect stings—not to the first sting, usually, but to subsequent ones. And the response may not be confined to stings by wasps, hornets, yellow jackets, and other barbed enemies. There is reason to believe that bites by black flies, fleas, ticks and various mites may also cause a reaction. If you think that your dog shows signs of being sensitive to any of these, you should discuss the problem with your veterinarian.

THE EYES

. . . it has often been said, are windows to a dog's body, and that is a medical fact as well as poetic fancy. Symptoms of scores of diseases are reflected in altered conditions of the eyes, and by a careful evaluation of these signs a veterinarian can often gather a vast amount of information about the general state of the dog's health. And the older the dog, the more revealing these windows to the body become.

The range and variety of these symptomatic clues is unbelievably wide. Jaundice is a primary sign of liver disease and one of the first places it becomes obvious is in the eyes. Paleness in the conjunctiva (the mucous membrane lining the inner surface of the eyelid) and an excessive brightness in the whites of the eyes are signs of anemia. Allergies are often responsible for discharges from the eyes. Twitching of the eyes may be evidence of a stroke or a concussion or of a problem in the middle ear. When an old dog is suffering from chronic nephritis, the blood vessels in the retina often show signs of hemorrhage. A rapid whitening of the lens and the appearance of cataracts is commonly linked to sugar diabetes. Conjunctivitis is sometimes an indication of a sinus problem, and other types of eye inflammation may be caused by an infection of the throat or tonsils. And signs of a whole host of infectious diseases, from distemper and hepatitis to tetanus and septicemia are reflected in changes in the dog's eyes.

From this it must be evident that eye problems are seldom what they seem, that home diagnosis and medication are reckless endangerment, that an eye condition can be properly treated only by correcting the cause—which is often remote and generally unsuspected by the owner. There are, of course, also specific disorders of the eye itself, but they too are difficult for the layman to identify and in most cases impossible for him to treat. An eye problem, in short, is almost always a problem for the veterinarian.

The *eyelids* are subject to a variety of ills and injuries. They are exceedingly sensitive and when they itch or burn the dog will often paw at them until the lids and sometimes the whole eye becomes inflamed. Mange may appear on the lids or a skin fungus may creep down over them. Both must be treated with great care and only with medications which will not injure the eye. Warts sometimes appear either on or under the lid and these, of course, cause the dog great discomfort. With old dogs it is not uncommon for eyelids to roll inward so that the lashes rub against the eyeball. Both of these last conditions can be—and generally must be—corrected by surgery.

Conjunctivitis, an inflammation of the skin layer under the lids and around the eye, is a catchall term for a condition of many types and many causes. In addition to being a common symptom of diseases elsewhere in the body, it can be the result of cuts, scratches, and foreign bodies such as weed seeds, dust, sand, and the like. It can also be caused by bites and bee stings. Unless the irritating substance is removed promptly, the conjunctiva may become so inflamed that the eye will swell shut and the membrane protrude. It is a painful condition and can become a serious one. Even with treatment it is sometimes necessary to use a sedative or a local anesthetic to keep the dog from injuring the eye itself.

As the dog grows older a grayish tinge appears in the pupils of the eyes. Owners are often alarmed by the change in the appearance of the eyes, and it is not uncommon for them to assume that it is a cataract or a sign of some form of progressive blindness. It isn't. It is a perfectly normal change that occurs in all dogs, and, though there is a wide variation from dog to dog, the gray generally begins to be evident some time around the fifth or sixth year. It is caused by a change in the lens itself. In a young dog the lens is clear and transparent, but in older dogs it becomes cloudy. We still don't know what causes the change, but it always occurs—so reliably that it used to be thought (mistakenly) that an old dog's age could be accurately estimated by examining his eyes.

A *cataract,* which is also an opacity of the lens, is an entirely different matter. The light entering the eye is focused by the lens and when a cataract develops, the lens gradually turns opaque and eventually it may become so white that it excludes most if not all of the light. The causes are not yet definitely known, but as I have said before, cataracts are often associated with certain diseases, notably diabetes. I suspect, too, that in many cases they are hereditary. They occur more frequently in old dogs than in young ones, but the onset may come at any age and cataracts are by no means unheard of in dogs only three or four years old. Cataracts usually, but not always, affect both eyes, but they may develop at different rates and the vision of one eye is often much more restricted than that of the other. Cataracts are generally progressive, but that is not an invariable rule, and occasionally their development slows down or stops altogether while the dog still has considerable vision in one or both eyes. And some cataracts never become so dense that they exclude all light and cause total blindness.

The surgical removal of a cataract from a human eye is a delicate but common operation today, and the same kind of surgery is also feasible with dogs. Indeed, it is being frequently performed in recent years. It is not uncommon for cataracts to cause a partial loss of vision, but as I have said earlier, an old dog accommodates remarkably well even when his sight is greatly diminished. The loss of the sight of one eye—or its removal—seems neither to hamper nor disturb a dog greatly, and many an old fellow continues to get around surprisingly well even though when tested he appears to be almost blind. It is difficult for an owner to believe, but the fact is that in an old dog impaired vision or even total blindness is not nearly the disaster that it is in a human being.

Glaucoma, which is sometimes inherited but may have other causes as well, is the result of an increase in the pressure of the fluid in the eye and the consequent enlargement of the eyeball. As the condition grows more severe, the eyes become distended, often so painfully that the dog must be given prompt attention and relief. Glaucoma is one of the most common causes of blindness in dogs and, unhappily, there is as yet no very effective treatment for it except surgery. Usually both eyes are involved, but occasionally the disease affects only one. In such cases, if the condition cannot be corrected either by surgery or treatment, the diseased eye should be removed, since if it isn't the other is likely to be affected also. The operation does not greatly handicap the dog, nor does it scar and disfigure him nearly as badly as most owners fear that it will. The lid is closed and, particularly with breeds with long coats, the hair around the eye covers the area so that at a glance few people even notice that the dog has lost an eye.

There are, of course, many other conditions which affect the eyes—injuries and diseases involving every part from the cornea and the lens to the retina and the optic nerve. But fortunately they are relatively rare—so rare that they have no place in a book of this sort.

The Ears

. . . are complicated (and to the anatomist, beautiful) instruments exquisitely designed to capture sound waves and almost miraculously to translate them into meaningful impulses that can be carried to the brain by the auditory nerves. Surely the ear is one of the great marvels of this world.

But to ignore the marvel and get to the business—the ear consists of three parts: the external ear, which is the flap and the canal leading to the eardrum; the middle ear, which is the cavity behind the drum that contains three delicate bones which vibrate in response to changing pressure and a tube (the Eustachian tube) which connects to the throat; and the inner ear, which houses the terminals of the nerves leading to the brain and the semicircular canals which control equilibrium.

For all its complexity, there are few life-threatening problems associated with the ear. But with old dogs the worrisome, nuisance problems are many and comparatively frequent.

Ear canker (an unfortunate name), is an infection of the canal of the external ear, and one of the most common. It sometimes has a very sudden onset, and often the first clue you get is that the dog's ears have become so tender that he whimpers or turns his head away when you scratch them. A few days later you are likely to notice a foul odor about his ears (a "cheesy" smell, it is sometimes called) and you may discover that he has a "soupy" ear with a good deal of discharge. The dog may hold his head a bit to one side and repeatedly (but very gingerly) scratch his ear with a back foot. The condition should be promptly treated by flushing the wax and foul discharge from the ear and applying medication appropriate for the particular kind of infection that is present. That must be done carefully and thoroughly and it is not a job that most owners can handle. Treatment is usually effective, but in stubborn cases it is sometimes necessary to grow cultures to identify the causative agent and treatment must be continued for a considerable time.

The symptoms of *ear mites* are often confused with those caused by canker. But the condition is entirely different. The problem is not an infection but an irritation caused by an infestation of tiny insects that are barely visible. The mites enter the ear canal and reproduce there at a great rate. Even a few of the pests will cause such severe itching that the dog will scratch incessantly and spend hours rubbing his ears along the rug or in the grass. There are slow home remedies—liberal amounts of mineral oil in the canal every day for two or three weeks—but a veterinarian can easily provide a quicker and more effective medication.

The latter solution would seem to be the sensible one —particularly since many owners seem to have remarkable ideas of what ear mites really are. Some have outrageous misconceptions. I'd be embarrassed to tell you how many solid and seemingly knowledgeable clients of mine have brought old dogs to the office and solemnly announced, "Doc, I'm afraid he's got those damned ear mice again."

When dogs with long ears shake their heads vigorously, the tips of their ears move with great speed and if they strike a solid object, the fragile veins are sometimes ruptured. Even determined, hard scratching with a hind foot can cause such an injury. Though there may be no external bleeding, the blood sometimes collects in a pocket, a *hematoma,* under the skin. In time the blood is generally reabsorbed, but nevertheless these hematomas should be attended to. If they are not treated, the skin is likly to thicken and discolor and to leave an ugly puckered area, often called a "potato chip" ear.

Warts often develop on or in an old dog's ears, sometimes even deep within the external canal. If there are many or if they continue to grow, they set up an irritation that constantly distresses the dog. And if they block the canal, the problem can easily develop into a generalized ear infection. They should, of course, be removed before that can happen. Furthermore, malignancies which look much like common warts are not uncommon in the ear. And with them the only hope of saving the dog lies in early and complete removal.

A minor problem, but a frequent nuisance, is the growth of excessive amounts of hair in the ear. Some breeds—the Poodle first among them—are prone to this small affliction. Aside from being unsightly, a wad of hair in an ear can inhibit the circulation of air in the canal and thus increase the likelihood of infections and other ear problems. Most groomers make it a practice to remove some of the hair, but if your dog isn't getting regular cosmetic attention, you can—without seriously distressing the old dog—pluck out a little of the hair with your fingers from time to time.

All dogs have some loss of hearing as they grow older, and by and large they accept the loss and adjust to it gracefully and well. Too well, sometimes, for owners often fail to realize how seriously the dog's hearing has been impaired and allow him to be dangerously exposed to accidents.

The aging process itself accounts for much of the dog's loss of hearing. All of his senses are dulled by age—scent excepted—and though the deterioration probably begins fairly early, it is generally not noticeable until the dog gets into his middle years. Here again genetic factors seem to make a decisive difference. Some breeds and some strains clearly have minor hearing problems sooner and more often than others do and they also tend to become deaf more frequently than dogs usually do. Sometimes there may be an almost total loss of hearing in one ear while the other is scarcely affected, and this too seems to run in certain lines. And since we know so little about these genetically controlled conditions, it is not surprising that there is little that we can do about them.

But deafness is also caused by infections, diseases, and injuries, and proper treatment will often prevent the loss of hearing and even improve hearing that has long been impaired. Anything that physically blocks the external canal—such as the growths mentioned above—can greatly diminish hearing, and the removal of these obstructions often results in a startling improvement. Even wax that has been allowed to harden and become impacted will cause partial deafness, and many a veterinarian has greatly improved his standing with an owner simply by clearing the gunk out of his dog's ears.

The inner ear is susceptible to infections which are not only extremely painful but also often permanently damage the dog's hearing. Such infections were once difficult to treat, but with the use of antibiotics they can now be controlled much more quickly and surely. They should be treated vigorously not only because of the pain and the immediate danger, but also because of the damage which may become evident only much later.

It is true that an old dog is often condemned to bear the lingering consequences of diseases and injuries that he suffered when he was young. And in many such cases the damage that has been done cannot be undone or repaired. But it often happens that the growing deafness which an owner associates with an old illness and assumes is beyond repair is actually a condition that *can,* in fact, be treated.

It may be that your old dog is growing deaf simply because he is growing old. But there may be other reasons. Nothing can be lost by discussing the problem with your veterinarian.

Parasites

. . . many people think, are problems only for pups and young dogs. But unfortunately they are wrong, for old Hector is susceptible to parasites—internal and external—all the days of his life. It is a dangerous mistake to assume that your dog has reached an age when he is past the danger of picking up parasites. He hasn't.

Old dogs do sometimes seem to develop a resistance of some sort to parasites. This has been observed particularly with roundworms and it may also be true to a lesser extent with other types of intestinal worms. But so far as I know the assumption that such resistance does develop is based on vague general impressions and has never been conclusively demonstrated by a controlled scientific study. At best it is true only of *some* dogs and whatever difference there is between young and old dogs may be due to factors other than a developing immunity.

Certainly there are many more obvious reasons why some dogs are more likely than others to get parasites. There are, it seems, innate differences between dogs in habits of cleanliness. Some seem predisposed to smell or lick or even taste every malodorous bit they find in the grass or gutter, and no matter how vigorously their owners scold and tug at their leashes, the dogs persist in their search for whatever is forbidden and untouchable. Others are dainty to the point of being meticulous. They seem almost to tiptoe around any unpleasantness they find in their way. Why the difference? I don't know. And I suppose that once again we will have to attribute it to some unknown genetic factor. But there can be no doubt that the dainty dog has a far lower incidence of intestinal parasites than the indiscriminate licker.

And today no one can be surprised that the local environment itself is a major factor in parasitic infestations. It is obvious that if you live in a city with a large dog population, your dog is more likely to have worms than if you live in a country hideaway. On the streets there are bound to be more dogs, more stools, more worm eggs —and more worms in Hector's intestines.

Tapeworms are not the most common of the intestinal parasites. But these eighteen-inch monsters (the most common type) are surely the most shocking to owners and the most readily identified. The segments from which the worms develop can easily be seen on a freshly passed stool. They look like motorized grains of rice, white to off-white in color, which appear to alternately elongate and shrink up as they move. Sometimes these creeping segments cause an itchy bottom which makes the old dog drag his rear across the rug or the grass. Only rarely do tapeworms create any digestive disturbance—and they don't really cause starvation—but they do give off toxins which poison the dog's system. There are patent medicines advertised as cures, of course. But the safe and effective remedies are available only on prescription. They work quickly and well, and presumably that is what you want and will get for Hector.

Hookworms and *whipworms,* however, do cause serious digestive problems. And beyond that, in heavy infestations they become a threat to the dog's life. Veterinarians think that in some parts of the United States—the warmer parts—hookworms kill more dogs than any other intestinal parasite. In the northern areas, I think, whipworms are more lethal. But wherever you live, you should realize that both are more than unpleasant visitations. They are real threats.

Hookworms—of which there are several varieties—are half-inch bloodsuckers which attach themselves to the lining of the intestines. I don't know who made the precise calculations, but some texts say that each adult hookworm causes the loss of one cc. of blood—a thimbleful—every week. If that is true, 100 hookworms—which is not a heavy infestation—would account for 100 cc.s of blood a week, and there are few dogs, old or young, that can afford such a loss for very long. The microscopic eggs in the stools need warmth to develop, which is why hookworms are a summertime threat in the North but a year-around plague in the South. The larvae are usually ingested through the mouth, but they can bore through the skin and can also be breathed in with dust or sniffed up from the ground. And that makes the hookworm a most persistent and ubiquitous menace wherever it is.

The whipworm—longer and thinner than the hookworm and equally voracious—anchors itself either to the lining of the intestinal wall or the cecum. Unlike the hookworm, it does not feed on the animal's blood but on the nutrients in the intestines. Both types of worms may cause diarrhea with blood and mucous, but with a whipworm infestation the first half of the stool is often near normal and only the end is loose and bloody. In the final stage of an infestation, the stools are a mass of bloody mucous.

Hookworms and whipworms both go through a cycle of development beginning with microscopic eggs which are distributed in feces. You can greatly reduce the chances of infestation by keeping the dog's run as clean and free of breeding material as possible. But there is no feasible way to completely protect the dog from exposure. Nor can you by simple observation know when infestation has begun. The safe and simple way to protect the dog is to have your veterinarian do periodic examinations of the dog's stools so that the worms can be destroyed before they begin to weaken the old dog or cause severe anemia. The treatment may be quick and easy. But not always. In some cases it must be repeated several times. The caution given above about the use of over-the-counter remedies applies here too. The veterinarian who makes the fecal examination can prescribe a more effective medication than the patent medicines on the market.

There are other internal parasites—esophageal worms, kidney worms, lung worms—but they are relatively uncommon in old dogs. If your dog does happen to pick up any of these, the chances are that they will be discovered only by the veterinarian in the course of a regular checkup. And he will treat them.

But one of the internal parasites which used to be a rarity in most of the United States must now be given serious attention. *Heartworms* are being reported almost everywhere today. Even in New England, where they were almost unknown twenty-five or thirty years ago, they have become a common problem. And the change is not merely the result of more careful diagnosis or better reporting. Veterinarians have long made it a practice to do postmortems whenever they were permitted, and it is only in recent years that heartworms have been discovered in large numbers of cases. The incidence *is* increasing rapidly. Some combination of circumstances or events has caused the extraordinary proliferation of this parasite, and there is no evident reason to hope that it will slow down. On the contrary, it is likely to spread even more widely. The mosquito is the infecting agent, and I suspect that heartworms will soon be a major threat in all areas where mosquitoes are a problem.

Both diagnosis and treatment are difficult. Heartworms live, mature, and reproduce in the blood in the right side of the heart. They are repulsive creatures. The adult females grow to be as much as fourteen inches long and perhaps one-sixteenth of an inch in diameter, the males to ten inches. The mature female produces an enormous number of microfilaria—up to two thousand every twenty-four hours—and these "wigglers" are dispersed throughout the bloodstream. When a female mosquito bites an infested dog, some of these wigglers are sucked up in the drop or so of blood she draws through her proboscis. (And a curious and unexplained thing about that is that though by analysis there may be no more than three or four wigglers in two cc.s of blood, the mosquito may draw six or eight of them in the single drop of blood she extracts.) The infective larvae develop in the mosquito and some of them are deposited with the secretions around her drilling mechanism when she bites another dog. They enter the wound, find their way through the bloodstream to the dog's right ventricle, mature and begin the reproductive cycle all over again. It's a long process. Prolific as the heartworms are, it takes at least five months and perhaps longer to produce enough larvae for the veterinarian to be able to make a positive diagnosis.

Destroying a mass of worms in a dog's heart is a delicate business. When you consider that a small blood clot in the coronary artery is enough to kill a human being, it seems almost impossible that a dog could survive with twenty-five or more of these foot-long worms dead in his heart. And yet, with proper care and medication nearly all dogs with heartworms can be saved—all but about 5 percent of those treated.

But the treatment must be carefully planned and controlled. The number of wigglers in the blood is not a reliable indication of the size of the infestation, so an x-ray is often taken to determine the amount of enlargement the worms have caused. The veterinarian must also be certain that the organs that will be most severely stressed during the treatment—the heart, the liver, the kidneys—are functioning properly, and if any weaknesses are discovered, they must be corrected before the treatment is undertaken. The veterinarian then administers an arsenical compound intravenously four times over a two-day period. During that time the dog must be observed regularly for signs of any of several problems that may arise and be given immediate treatment should any of them occur.

The incidence of heartworms is alarming. But there is at least a hope that the preventive program now being used will prove fully effective. A new program involves giving the dog prescribed daily doses of an insect-inhibiting drug during the mosquito season. The drug seems to ward off the mosquitoes and prevent their biting. As this is written, the results seem most promising, and by the time you read it, they may have been fully confirmed. I suggest—I urge—that you ask your veterinarian to keep you informed about the results of research in this field.

External parasites are a fading problem. They are no longer a scourge to dogs and in general they are not nearly as insidious or dangerous as the internal parasites. But they do still exist, and if it has become easier to get them off the dog, it often seems that it is more difficult to get them out of the house.

Today *lice* are no more than a nuisance and almost a nuisance of the past. Only once or twice a year, perhaps, do I see a poor neglected old dog who is infested. Either lice are disappearing or all owners have learned how to prevent and destroy them. In either case it seems hardly worthwhile to discuss the life and nasty habits of the louse here. If your dog happens to fall in with bad company and become infested, your veterinarian—after he gets over his surprise—will be able to tell you in a minute how to end the problem.

These days I find that people are more troubled *about* lice than dogs are *by* lice. Not long ago a young couple brought in their dog just to ask me how they were to rid him of lice. They seemed so confident of his problem that I examined the animal with extra care—and found no signs of an infestation. "How do you know your dog has lice?" I asked cautiously. "Oh, we know all right," the woman said with some reluctance. "We caught them from him." I had to tell the young people that the louse that was troubling them could neither feed on the old dog nor be transmitted by him—that it was, in fact, a social problem shared solely by people. It was a brief but difficult lesson in entomology. The couple was amazed. The wife looked at the husband, the husband looked at the wife, the question of who got lice when and where hung in the air, and even the veterinarian was embarrassed.

But *fleas* are not fastidious. When times are hard the flea will feed on either man or beast, and to get rid of a heavy infestation of fleas in a house can be a major undertaking. The problem is that the flea eggs drop off the dog, incubate, hatch, molt, climb a little way up whatever is near, and hop onto the first warm body that passes. While they don't especially relish people, fleas are willing to sample a good ankle or make do with the children's tender skin until a tasty dog comes along. After the dog has had fleas for a while, eggs will have been deposited all over the premises, and they will be in all stages of development. You can wash the dog until every flea has perished in medicated suds, and before his coat has dried, he'll have as many as he had before the bath began. I have had people tell me that they have had to completely seal off their basements because the whole area was hopping. When things have reached that stage, bathing a dog merely prepares him nicely for a new crop of fleas waiting for their first meal. It will at least be necessary to spray the whole place repeatedly with a powerful insecticide, and you may have to have the premises fumigated. It is usually best, I think, to consult your veterinarian. He'll probably be able to help you solve your problem for less than you would have to pay a professional fumigator—the rewards of much study being what they are today.

That *ticks* are a tough problem is an understatement. One reason for that is that the large, gray female tick is capable of laying between five thousand and seven thousand eggs in a *week*—and virtually all of them hatch. They will develop almost anywhere. If your old dog has ticks in the wintertime, they are hatching in the house, and you have the same sort of problem that fleas create. The tick that feeds on Hector usually won't trouble you, but if you have had experience with the variety that likes people, you know how deviously ticks work. They cause no pain, no itching, no discomfort of any sort. The feeding ticks simply sit there engorging themselves endlessly until they become so large that you happen to see them or feel them. So it is with Hector, though he may sometimes develop a local inflammation, perhaps from the tick's saliva.

The plump, gray tick that you see on the dog is female—prettier and bigger than the male, who apparently does not feed on the dog at all but merely attaches himself to the skin nearby and waits to perform his essential duties. You should look for the inconspicuous little fellow hiding in the hair near the big tick and destroy him, too. Contrary to what everybody has been told, you don't have to dab each tick with turpentine or gasoline before you remove it. Since it does not bury its head in the skin but uses only its mouth parts to suck blood, you can't leave the head embedded under the surface when you pull the tick off. Still, you shouldn't simply cut the tick off flush with the surface since the mouth parts that remain may cause unnecessary, lingering irritation.

What do you do when your dog keeps gathering ticks every time he goes out of the house? The procedure is primitive but effective. First you pick off the ticks daily and carefully, making certain that you've got them all and have inspected such hiding places as the spaces between the toes, top and bottom. And you destroy them—which, you will discover, is not as easy as it sounds. They are tough. If you have trouble disposing of them, you can always drop them into a container of water saturated with a detergent.

And then, if they have invaded the house, you have the task of cleaning up the area where the eggs are incubating. That is a job that has to be done with the same vigor and thoroughness that is used to rid a house of fleas. Here again, instead of calling in a fumigator, you might do better to ask your veterinarian to recommend a safe and effective spray.

There is one other parasite, at least semiexternal, that should be mentioned. It is the so-called *nasal* or *lung mite*. Nasal mites are probably more common than we realize since they crawl out of the dog's nostrils and are either brushed off or licked off before the owner notices them. They are barely visible and look like no more than traveling bits of dandruff or perhaps some tiny white aphidlike creatures that might have been picked up from the grass. If you have never heard that there are such things as nasal mites and if you don't always wear your glasses, you are unlikely to discover that your dog has them. And the veterinarian who is with your dog for only a few minutes now and then may never see him when the mites are abroad and visible. So if the dog begins to sneeze more than usual and for no apparent reason and if he keeps rubbing his nose as though he has an itch that can't be scratched away, you have reason to suspect that he has nasal mites. Discovering the problem is the problem. Your veterinarian will take it from there.

Arthritis

. . . like all of the *-itis* ills in the catalog, is an inflammation rather than a disease as such, an inflammation of one or more of the joints. It is a vague and inclusive term that is commonly used and misued to cover dozens of painful conditions. I have been told that more than two hundred types of arthritis have been described in human beings and I suspect that in time veterinarians will identify as many kinds in dogs. Among old dogs, certainly, it is a major problem—one of the most common and in some ways one of the most distressing of the chronic ailments.

Owners often think that all forms of arthritis are progressive, excruciatingly painful, and eventually incapacitating. Fortunately, their fears are grossly exaggerated. It is true that among the many types there are those—some forms of osteoarthritis, for example—in which permanent bone changes takes place and the joint may be totally immobilized. But in the great majority of cases the ravages are far less severe, and the condition, though painful, never becomes totally destructive.

The first signs of arthritis often begin to appear when the dog is middle-aged—sometimes in his early middle age—though it is probable that the condition has been developing over a period of time. Generally the onset is gradual and the owner notices only that the dog sometimes has a little difficulty in getting up or seems to be a little stiff until he has moved around for a while. Occasionally the signs appear suddenly. The old dog comes in from what seems to be a light session of exercise, but after a rest one leg has become almost immobilized, and the dog is forced to hobble around on three. The difficulty is often localized in a single joint, and veterinarians sometimes call it "football knee," since it involves the ligaments that athletes commonly have trouble with. The condition is treatable, and though it may require a good deal of rest and medication—and in severe cases, surgery—the damage usually can be repaired and the dog put back on four feet.

The less disabling types of arthritis which develop more slowly can also be treated, but for the most part the treatment is aimed at reducing the pain and keeping the animal as comfortable and mobile as possible. Since we don't know what causes this nasty assortment of ills—injuries, infections, viruses, old age, or simply the degeneration of joint tissue have all been blamed—the medications generally used are intended to *alleviate* rather than to *cure*. Happily there are many forms of arthritis which never become more than mildly discomforting. And for those that continue to develop and in time threaten to become disabling we now have a sequence of drugs which makes it possible to keep a dog ambulatory much longer than we once could.

Mild and intermittent cases of arthritis can often be substantially eased simply by making certain that the dog has dry, warm quarters to sleep in and by providing a somewhat softer bed than he has been used to. I have known many instances in which arthritic pains were greatly relieved by fitting the dog's bed with a heating pad—kept at a very low heat and installed with the proper precautions.

And aspirin is still the drug of choice in many cases. Indeed, aspirin alone is often all that old Hector needs to see him through a painful bout of arthritis that if left untreated would have kept him hobbling for days or weeks. But don't just dose him with the stuff. Find out from your veterinarian how much the dog should get at what intervals.

In difficult cases the cortisone-like drugs—the steroids—are often the best and sometimes the only effective treatment. They produce remarkable results both when the arthritis affects only a local area and when it is more generalized. But the steroids generally have the same undesirable side effects with dogs as they do with people. They are usually prescribed only after other measures have failed and often they cannot be continued indefinitely at an effective level.

Though we still have no cure for arthritis, we have come a long way from the time when it was a lingering, chronic misery from which there was no escape. Today your veterinarian can almost always provide some degree of relief for an arthritic old dog and often he can devise some course of treatment that will keep the pain within tolerable limits for years and prevent the dog from ever becoming completely disabled.

Posterior Paralysis

. . . or *paraplegia,* is perhaps the cruelest of all the disabling afflictions. And it is, I think, the one most dreaded by owners.

The onset is generally calamitously sudden. And the symptoms—as every veterinarian who has taken those frantic midnight calls knows—are unmistakably clear. Just before bedtime, the owner reports, he gathered up the leash and called the old dog for his nightly turn around the block. But the dog didn't come, and the owner found him struggling to get out of his bed. Though he had appeared to be perfectly well only an hour or so before, he was suddenly unable to move the back part of his body. When the owner picked him up and tried to stand him on his feet, he sagged to the floor. His hind legs were completely paralyzed.

The owner finds it hard to believe that such a change could occur in a few minutes, while the dog was resting or asleep. And it probably didn't. More likely there had been a slow, progressive deterioration in the spine, and just before the dog lay down some slight stress had snapped the weakest link and an intervertebral disc had given way. The accident caused acute inflammation and swelling, and pressure was put on the spinal column. By the time the poor old dog tried to get up, paralysis had set in, and he was unable to move any part of his body beyond the pressure point.

Paraplegia is surely one of the most heartbreaking situations an owner ever has to face. The dog—the fore part—appears to be quite normal. He is responsive, he usually eats well, and often he seems to be not so much in pain as mystified by what has happened to him. But from the area of involvement down his body has nearly or completely ceased to function.

In a younger dog—and occasionally in a very strong old dog—it may be possible to do something to relieve the pressure and repair the damage surgically. But under the best of circumstances, it is a difficult, risky operation and the odds vary with the degree of damage. In most cases the only thing to do is to wait and hope that the damage has not been so severe that the paralysis is permanent and irreversible. During that time—and a week will generally tell the story—the veterinarian will administer drugs to ease the pain. If the dog begins to show signs of movement in his hindquarters within a few days, there may be hope. With prolonged treatment—and with the most demanding nursing care an owner can ever be expected to give—the dog may recover sufficiently to move about and perform the necessary bodily functions. But rarely, if ever, will there be anything like a full recovery. In nearly half of the cases, tragically, the dog does not regain the use of the lower body, and euthanasia becomes the only humane solution.

Anemia

. . . is basically a lack of hemoglobin (and consequently, of oxygen) in the blood. It can be caused either by too little blood in the system or by too few red cells in the blood. That much is clear and simple—and it is about all that *is* simple about anemia.

The symptoms are familiar. The dog—often quite suddenly—seems to lose energy, interest, and stamina. He becomes tired and droopy. He may continue to eat and drink as usual, but he is reluctant even to get up and move about. When he does, he seems weary unto death and he may even stumble as he goes. All of this you can easily see. When you take him to be examined, the veterinarian will point out that the tissue around the eyes has a bleached look. The gums are pale. When they are pressed above the canine teeth, they turn white and the pink color is very slow to return after the pressure is released.

The chief difficulty with anemia comes in discovering what is causing the condition. There are scores of possible causes. Red blood cells are produced in the bone marrow—half a million cells per *second* in a normal dog—and the cells live for about one hundred days. But not until the count falls 50 percent below normal do signs appear, and even then it takes extremely delicate tests to show whether a sufficient number of cells are being produced. Or the condition could be caused by a shortage of hemoglobin. That could be caused by a lack of iron in the diet. Or by the failure of the body to utilize it properly. The anemia could be the result of slow internal bleeding. A heavy infestation of hookworms often and easily draws enough blood to make a dog anemic. Toxins produced by any number of diseases can create an anemic condition. Or the mechanism which regulates the proportion of red and white cells in the blood may have gone askew. And these are only a sampling of the possible causes.

Sometimes, of course, the cause or causes of anemia are evident. But more often they aren't. And when they are unusual or obscure, the veterinarian may have to make a wearisome series of laboratory tests before he can make a diagnosis and begin treatment.

The cure for the cause of the anemia is the cure for the

anemia. Treatment is as varied as the causes. It is sometimes prolonged, but it is generally effective and seldom difficult.

It is the search that wears down the veterinarian and strains his intuitive powers.

Contagious Diseases

. . . are not respecters of old age. Old dogs are generally not as vulnerable to them as pups and young dogs—partly, perhaps, because they sometimes develop a resistance or immunity of sorts, but also, I suspect, simply because they don't get around as much and are therefore exposed less. But make no foolish mistakes. Old Hector can catch anything that is contagious.

There are only four major contagious diseases, I think, which owners of old dogs need be concerned about. Two of them—infectious canine hepatitis and leptospirosis—have been discussed earlier in this section because they affect the liver and its functions. The other two—rabies and distemper—are both virus infections and both have been among the most devastating diseases of dogdom.

Today no dog should ever get any of these four diseases. For all of them there are now reliable vaccines which when properly administered insure dependable immunity. The true cause of any of them is now simply the owner's neglect.

Rabies—hydrophobia in the old days—was a common horror until Pasteur demonstrated the effectiveness of inoculation. Less than a century ago the fear of rabies was so pervasive that when an outbreak occurred in New York City a bounty was offered to any urchin who found a dog loose in the street and brought him in for slaughter. Rabies was a horrible disease and the primitive measures taken to prevent its spread were almost as horrible.

In rabies the bite of an infected animal introduces the virus to the system, and from the wound it travels along the nerves until it reaches the brain. It moves slowly in the nerve tissue and the onset of the disease itself ranges from three weeks after the bite when it is near the brain to as much as three months later when the wound is in the extremities. Contrary to what most people believe, the animal does not always become a howling, raving beast. It may go into a period of profound depression, which is later followed by hysteria, convulsion, and the eventual paralysis and death.

When regulations requiring the inoculation of dogs were widely instituted, the incidence of rabies declined dramatically. In New England rabies is now a rarity, and in my own state of Connecticut there has not been a single reported case in dogs in more than twenty-five years. But rabies has not been wiped out. It is still a threat throughout much of the United States, particularly in the South. Worse, the virus affects all warm-blooded animals, and in recent years rabies has been on the increase in many species. The skunk is thought to be the chief carrier of the virus today, but the reports of outbreaks of the disease in foxes, coyotes, raccoons, and bats have also been alarming.

Without exceptions, all dogs—even *your* old dog—should be inoculated. In the past the procedure was to give the dog his first injection before he was a year old, another when he became a year old, and one each year thereafter. Today, however, there are a number of variations to this schedule, depending upon the type of vaccine that is used.

Distemper is an old-fashioned term once used to describe what we now know to be a whole complex of diseases. The specific virus disease is loathsome and, as is true with most virus diseases, there is no medicine with which it can effectively be treated. The only defense your dog has is prevention. But that is all that he needs. The vaccine now in use provides reliable immunity.

Carré distemper, which once killed dogs by the thousands every year, is a disease which attacks all of the mucous membranes—in the eyes, the nose, the mouth, the intestines, the genitals, and many glands. The dog's nose becomes caked with a thick, stringy discharge, he coughs and gags, he is nauseated and giddy, he develops a foul diarrhea and later severe dehydration. And this disgusting disease may ravage the dog for a month or more until at last he dies twitching or in convulsions.

No one who has ever seen a dog with distemper is likely to neglect having his own dog properly inoculated. But not everybody has seen or knows.

Distemper inoculations can now be given in a number of different sequences. The thing for you to remember is that your dog has to have continued protection during his old age, and you must rely on your veterinarian to set up a schedule that will provide it.

Panic-Button Problems

And always—there are the emergencies.

You have been warned—endlessly, properly, here and elsewhere—that it is impossible for you to develop the skills and experience necessary to interpret contradictory and misleading symptoms that often baffle even the most experienced practitioner, that diagnosis and treatment are for your veterinarian and not for you.

True . . . all true.

And now, with equal reason and with equal severity, you are also warned that there are *some* symptoms you must be able to recognize and evaluate without hesitation and without question—that in emergency situations the failure to identify these symptoms promptly may well endanger your dog's life.

And that, too, is true.

Nothing, I suppose, would be of more use to an owner than a good reliable list of certified emergencies with the symptoms by which he could invariably recognize them. But emergencies don't come in neat categories, and their urgency and severity depend always on a host of variables of time and circumstance. And unfortunately there is no handy do-and-don't checklist to make it easy to handle them when they do occur.

What can you do about these panic-button problems? Can you be prepared to handle them when they happen?

Yes—to some degree you can. Nobody is ever fully prepared for an emergency. But by the same token nobody should be so ill prepared that he is completely unhinged when these life-threatening emergencies do arise. Usually there is little that you yourself will be able to do for the dog, but if you are aware of the usual symptoms of the common acute and critical illnesses, if you understand that immediate and intensive care is often the only hope in situations of this sort, you will be able to act effectively to help your dog through those first crucial hours of a crisis.

Most owners are overly reluctant to call a veterinarian outside his regular office hours. And it is indeed an imposition to rouse him to ask advice about some routine matter that could just as well wait until morning. But it is totally unforgivable to let your dog pass the point of no return simply because you don't recognize the seriousness of his symptoms or because you are unwilling to disturb your veterinarian's rest at three o'clock in the morning.

It is always hard to know what you can or will or should do in a moment of crisis. It seems to me that you can best prepare for that time by making up your mind here and now that if you find yourself in a situation where you don't know whether a condition is a true emergency or not, you will wisely and prudently assume that it is. If it turns out that it is not an emergency, your veterinarian will have been deprived of a little sleep that he had counted on. But if it *is* a panic-button situation and you sit it out until morning, you may have lost a dog.

There is no home guide to emergencies. You do what you can to familiarize yourself with the danger signals,

Panic-Button Chart

	Weight loss	Blood in urine	Discharge–nose and eyes	Excess urination–frequency	Hair loss	Excess thirst	*Fainting	*Problem urinating	*Jaundice	*Coma	Nervousness	Personality change	*Convulsions
Heart Disease													
Kidney Disease	●			●		●				●			●
Liver Disease									●				
Pancreatitis											●		
Prostatitis													
Heartworm	●												
Hypothyroidism													
Diabetes (sugar)	●			●		●				●			
Diabetes insipidus				●	●	●							
Leptospirosis			●						●				
Hypoglycemia										●	●		●
Stroke										●	●	●	
Distemper	●		●									●	●
Rabies										●	●	●	
Tetanus										●	●		
Kidney Stones		●				●							
Bladder Stones		●		●				●					
Shock										●			
Arthritis													
Epilepsy											●		●
Adrenal Insufficiency				●	●	●							
Concussion										●	●		
Cystitis				●				●					
Bronchitis													
Anemia							●						
Pyometra													

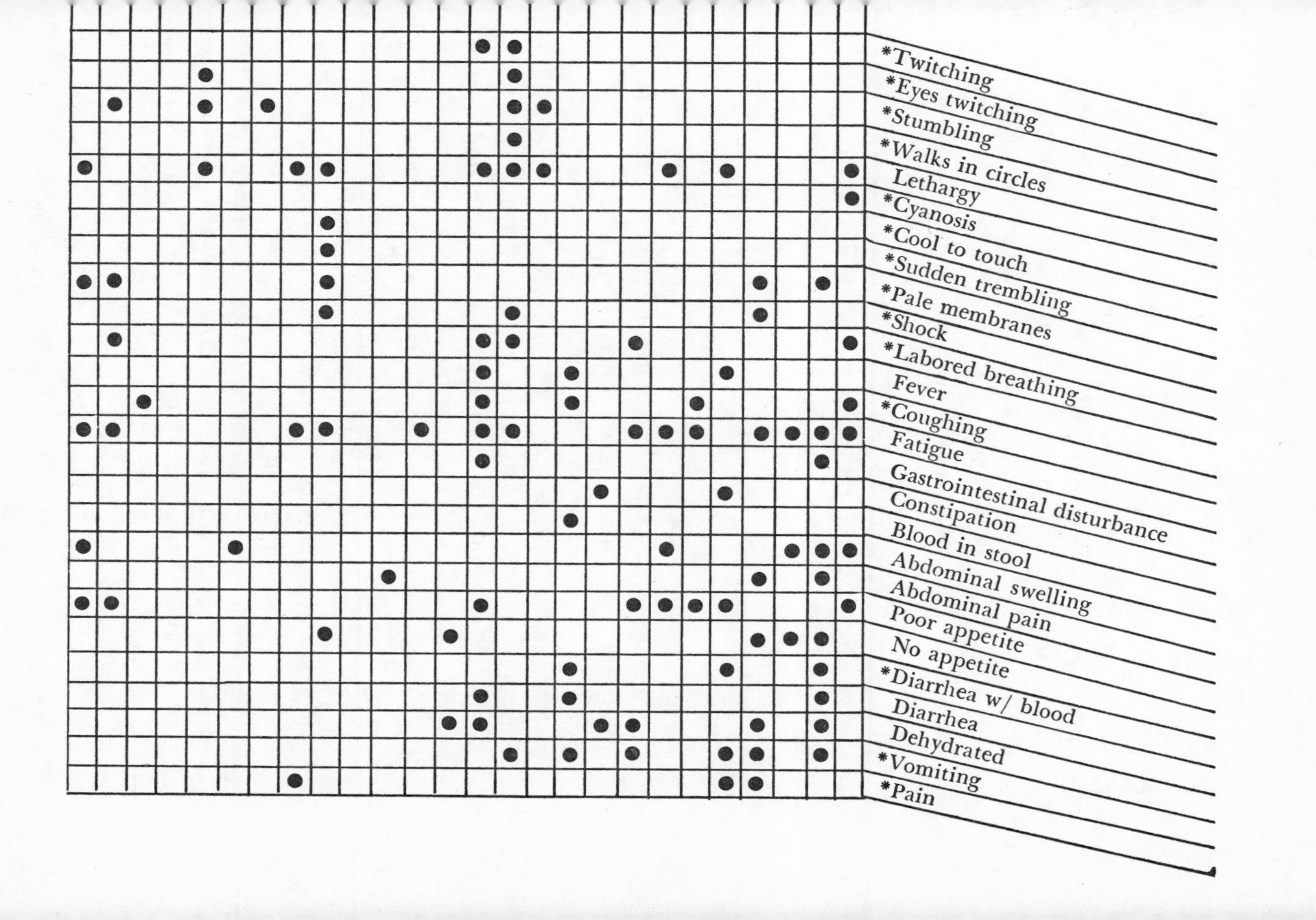

*Twitching														●	●											
*Eyes twitching					●										●											
*Stumbling		●			●		●								●	●										
*Walks in circles															●											
Lethargy	●				●			●	●					●	●	●				●		●				●
*Cyanosis																										●
*Cool to touch									●																	
*Sudden trembling									●																	
*Pale membranes	●	●							●														●		●	
*Shock									●						●								●			
*Labored breathing		●												●	●				●							●
Fever														●			●					●				
*Coughing			●											●			●				●					●
Fatigue	●	●						●	●			●		●	●				●	●	●		●	●	●	●
Gastrointestinal disturbance														●											●	
Constipation																		●				●				
Blood in stool																	●									
Abdominal swelling	●					●														●				●	●	●
Abdominal pain											●												●		●	
Poor appetite	●	●												●					●	●	●	●				●
No appetite									●				●										●	●	●	
*Diarrhea w/ blood																	●					●			●	
Diarrhea														●			●								●	
Dehydrated													●	●				●	●				●		●	
*Vomiting															●		●		●			●	●		●	
*Pain								●														●	●			

and your veterinarian does what he can to help you to recognize the signs of the most common problems. I have found that a brief chart of symptoms and the illnesses associated with them is useful and helpful for owners. The one reproduced here is inadequate, as all such charts are, and it is otherwise unsatisfactory in a number of ways. Worse, if the reader should be foolish enough to think that he could use it to arrive at a home dignosis, it could be a fatally dangerous tool. But if it is used sensibly, it does have some value. It lists a number of common conditions which in their acute forms are real emergencies. It indicates the pattern of symptoms commonly associated with these conditions. It alerts the owner to certain less obvious but significant signs that he might otherwise overlook. It serves as a checklist to prepare the owner for some of the over-the-phone questions which the veterinarian must ask before he can have even a preliminary opinion of the severity of the dog's problem.

The chart is certainly a most unreliable diagnostic guide. Its usefulness depends heavily on the perception and good judgment of the owner himself and on his ability to report what he sees accurately and completely. But it does offer a method—simple as it is—for organizing the information in some useful way. I offer it here, not because it is good, but because the alternative is nothing.

The symptoms included are of the most obvious sort—those that any observant owner should be able to recognize easily and surely. Those commonly associated with emergency situations are marked with an asterisk, and the appearance of any of these signs should be taken as an indication that a potentially dangerous condition may exist. The severity of the symptoms, the way they are grouped under the conditions listed, the frequency of their occurrence—all these are important, of course, and all must be properly evaluated by the veterinarian.

This is not a diagnostic chart. And it provides no information at all about the treatment your dog may need in an emergency. That is for your veterinarian to decide. It is no more than a simplified guide to some of the signs often associated with the common emergency situations. It is intended to do one thing only—to alert you to the fact that your dog may have difficulties that demand immediate attention. But if you understand its purpose and if you use it intelligently, it may prove to be the most important page in this book. It may be the means of saving your dog's life.

IX
Food: The Lethal Indulgence

It can't be overstated: Every year thousands—hundreds of thousands—of good old dogs are killed by their owners, by decent, gentle, kindly, concerned people who go on loving and feeding and overfeeding and fattening their dogs until they kill them.

Oscar Wilde wrote of the cruelty of friends who kill with a look, a kiss, or a word. In the dog's world the most lethal weapon is none of these. It is food. Too much food.

It is not *some,* and not even *many* owners who overfeed their dogs. It is almost *all* owners. And they overfeed enormously. Their dogs are not a little too fat, or somewhat overweight. They are grossly overweight—obese. I believe that half of the old dogs I see weigh half again as much as they should. And it is not unusual—indeed, it is common—to have an unconcerned owner bring in a waddling dog that scales in at twice his proper weight.

Fat kills dogs just as it kills people—as surely, as insidiously and for the same reasons. Nobody needs to be told again that excess weight burdens the body, that it causes excessive fatigue and shortness of breath, that it crowds the organs and interferes with their functions, that it dangerously increases the demands on the heart, that it overloads the joints and muscles, that it is associated with conditions such as diabetes and diseases of the kidneys and gallbladder, that it greatly increases the problems and risks in surgery. In study after study it has been demonstrated that obesity is a cause of death or, with other conditions, a contributing factor.

Owners know that fat kills. But still they continue to overfeed and fatten and destroy their dogs. Why?

There are no *reasons* to overfeed a dog. There are only excuses. And justifications. But of these there are an incredible number. Every veterinarian has heard scores of them. Dogs are being killed:

—Because owners think that it is "natural" for an old dog to get fat.

—Because they believe that a dog "knows" how much he should eat.

—Because owners don't know that as a dog grows older he needs less food than when he was younger.

—Because they think that if a dog used to eat a bowlful of food, that is the right amount for him now.

—Because they think that an "eager eater" is a healthy dog. If he eats well (much), he *is* well. If he eats less, there must be something wrong with him. Therefore, urge him to eat more.

—Because they "can't bear to see a dog hungry."

—Because they have so distorted the dog's taste that it is difficult to feed him sensibly.

—Because their concept of what a dog *should* or *must* have is a mass of misconceptions—myths, fallacies, and advertising slogans.

—Because food is love, and more food is *more* love—given and received.

Fat dogs are the veterinarian's most common, most persistent, and most difficult problem. He can relieve a dog that is in pain. He can treat a dog that is desperately sick and see him recover. He can mend a dog that has been broken and injured. But the overweight dog is a problem of a different sort. The veterinarian knows what can be done and what should be done. But in many cases, if not in most, he is powerless to do it. The endless procession goes on. The veterinarian's office becomes his purgatory—filled with fat dogs.

In matters related to diet and feeding, there are no problem dogs. There are only problem owners. And they are far more difficult to treat than their dogs. They are a bad group of good people who simply refuse to recognize the harm they are doing to their dogs with mindless kindness. They haven't noticed that their dogs are overweight. They don't know how much their dogs weigh—or how much they should weigh. They are regularly astonished to learn that much of what they *know* about feeding is clearly wrong. In the office they are usually agreeable listeners and willing converts to new and better ways. At home they harbor good intentions but they remain unwilling or unable to mend their ways and feed less—even though their dogs' lives depend on their making a change.

I don't know what can be done to jar these gentle executioners out of their apathy. Like every other veterinarian, I have tried in every way I can to warn them of the consequences. I threaten, insist, urge, cajole, plead, demand, beg and perform in other unseemly ways. And still the dogs grow fat. And sick.

It's a disgrace to have a fat dog. All you need to know to feed him properly and keep him in shape you can learn in fifteen minutes in your veterinarian's office. Not that animal nutrition is all that simple. It's a difficult and complex subject. But surely nobody thinks that it is necessary to become an authority on nutrition to feed a dog properly. The research has been done, the basic facts are known, and there is no need (and no possibility) for you to confirm them. All you need to know, actually, are the practical conclusions that have been drawn from these proven facts. That's all you need. That—and the good sense and discipline to feed your dog the right way instead of the easy way.

Feeding a dog properly is not difficult. But getting owners to rid themselves of the preconceptions and the misconceptions that prevent them from feeding as they should *is* difficult. The fallacies are ingrained, ingrown, and impacted. They have to be pried out.

The myth that is most firmly embedded, perhaps, is the peculiar notion that the more nearly the owner is able to duplicate the dog's "natural" diet the better. This is romanticized nonsense. The dog is not by any measure a *natural* wild animal. He is the first and most firmly domesticated of all of man's creatures and he has lived with people and adapted to their ways for millennia. If by the "natural" dog you mean an ancestral animal in its predomesticated stage, you must go back into the mists of the Paleolithic Age to some vaguely defined creature, possibly wolflike, about whom we actually know almost nothing. If our surmises are correct, his life was less than idyllic. It was a fang-and-claw struggle for existence and it is likely that only the strongest were able to escape sudden death and slow starvation long enough to reproduce. Perhaps the wolf living in the remotest parts of the world today faces similar hazards, but even he probably fares better now. He gorges himself on a kill (there are records of wolves who have ingested as much as thirty-five pounds at a time), eating the whole carcass, including the organs and their contents, in order to get the essential elements which flesh alone does not provide. Then he starves and hunts and kills again and survives if he is lucky. On the average, one pup in a litter survives the rigors of this life to reach maturity. And the so-called wild dogs who scavenge on the fringes of human society today fare no better. Your dog doesn't live the life of a wolf. And he is not a wild dog. If you fed him as they are fed, he would perish.

This fireside talk about a *natural* diet is rubbish.

Nevertheless, you must remember that even though the dog and his living conditions have changed immensely over the thousands of years of his close association with people, he does still retain some of the mechanisms which made it possible for him to survive in the wild. And not all of the physical characteristics your dog has carried over from history are useful and beneficial to him today. His stomach in some ways still resembles the stomach of an animal who ate fitfully, massively, and occasionally. It is far more capacious than it needs to be in an animal who lives securely in a household where good food is served regularly and reliably. That stomach gives him an appetite which causes him to eat much more than he actually needs. And when food is abundantly available, he will do just that.

A dog's body—like yours—has a "rainy day" conservation mechanism which once served as an essential aid to survival. When food was plentiful the unused excess was stored in fat that could later be converted to energy when there was no food to be had. But in these days of easy living in this country (and compared to the way dogs lived even half a century ago, these are truly lush times) hoarding fat is not a virtue. It would be far better for your dog—and easier for you—if it were possible to turn off this vestigial device. But it is resolutely and persistently automatic. Given the opportunity, your dog will eat more food than he needs to meet his current energy expenses. And inevitably he will become fat.

A dog that is overweight is overfed. You may, if you wish, say that you feed him little enough and that the real reason he is fat is that he doesn't get enough exercise. In a sense that is true. If he were very active, he would put on a little less weight. But you are not feeding a dog that runs all day and all night. You are feeding a dog that gets very little exercise—and you must feed him accordingly. At his age he is naturally less active than he once was, and even if he were willing to cooperate, you couldn't possibly work him enough to keep his weight down if you fed him all he would eat. If you jogged with him all day, *you* would lose weight. But he wouldn't.

The argument that it is natural for old dogs to get fat merits discussion. Briefly. It is *not* natural for old dogs to get fat. It *is* common. An old dog who is overfed does get fat. An old dog who is properly fed does not.

It is also alleged that Penelope is fat because she was spayed. That is not true either. Spaying has no effect, one way or the other, on a dog's weight. If Penelope is fat now, on the same diet she would be exactly as fat and not one pound slimmer if she had not been spayed.

And so it goes with all of the excuses. There is no need to refute them one by one. The plain and painful fact is that a healthy dog, whatever his age, gets fat for one reason and for one reason only. He is being overfed.

What your dog eats and how much he eats is entirely your responsibility. Through ages of association with man, the dog has become the most omnivorous of animals. He can, will, and in some corners of the world, does eat almost anything that is faintly digestible—fish, flesh, and bad red herring. And as long as he gets the necessary elements—carbohydrates, fats, proteins, minerals and vitamins—he will get along on almost any mixture that is provided, from trash fish with boiled potatoes to the carcass of a discarded mule.

A dog's tastes and eating habits are formed by his owner. If he has been raised on a commercial dehydrated dog food, he will eat it with pleasure and flourish on it for years. If he has been taught that garnished lamb chops and mint jelly are the proper food for him, he will expect to be served garnished lamb chops every day. With mint jelly. And if he has been bribed to bed every night with a bowl of ice cream, he will stay awake until he has it, even if he has to wait until you drive to town through a snowstorm to get it.

There is no law about what you may or can feed your

dog, and there is no limit to the amount of time, effort, and money that you can spend in providing food for him. I am tempted to say the effort and money you can *squander*. But that is a personal judgment. What is a pleasure for you is a pleasure for you, even though to others it may be a waste and an affront. You may feed your dog as you see fit, at least until it becomes necessary to allocate available calories to those in need throughout the world. I try to be tolerant of owners' foibles even though I come from New England, where babies are weaned on frugality and austerity. It is only when the way you feed your dog threatens to destroy him that I blow the whistle.

But I am willing to admit that I have no patience with the owner who has become the victim of the whimsical tastes he has himself created and nurtured in his dog. I don't want to hear complaints about the hours and love that it takes to prepare three exquisite meals a day for a dog—who, usually it seems, leaves the food uneaten and the love unrequited. I don't want to be asked again whether the eggs should be scrambled or poached, or how brown the sausage should be. And when I am told that the fat little dog on the table in front of me just *can't* lose weight, I explode.

"But I *have* to give her calf's liver sautéed in butter," says the distracted owner. "I *have* to. She won't eat anything else. She would die rather than eat that dog food!"

In a situation like that it is not hard for me to tell the owner the truth. No dog ever starved to death waiting for sautéed liver—not while there was anything edible available. In my most kindly fashion I explain that if the dog could find nothing else, she would eat watery gravy poured over sawdust. But believe me, I say gently, please believe me—*she will not starve*. But there may be a streak of meanness showing when I tell the owner that if the dog is getting only calf's liver in butter, she *will* starve. Even though she gets enough calories and minerals, she will develop a vitamin deficiency. It is called *avitaminosis.*

The little dog I have destroyed in the last paragraph is, of course, a straw dog. But cases of food deficiencies are common, and they are often created by owners who feed their dogs lavishly—on one food. I particularly remember two clients, a delightful couple whose sustaining pleasure in life came from raising Saint Bernards. They went to extraordinary lengths and expense to select and breed the finest of the breed in our part of the country. I know that every week at one time they were feeding their dogs $175 worth (Yes . . . yes . . .) of prime beef. And in addition, supplements and additives at what cost I don't know. For all of their efforts they were rewarded with more persistent trouble in raising pups than any breeder I knew. For years I was unable to persuade them to feed more sensibly, but finally (by begging a personal favor and urging the change in the interest of science) I convinced them to switch two brood bitches to an inexpensive commercial dog food. The mothers prospered astonishingly, *raising* litters of eleven and twelve pups while the meat eaters were raising an average of four. And when the rest of the dogs in the kennel were taken off the beef binge, the results were the same. To that couple I became a sage by recommending something that every owner should know. And if science was not really advanced by this one small demonstration of a well-known fact, some dozens of Saint Bernards had reason to be grateful.

You should feed your dog to support, sustain, and maintain his health. You can, if you are so minded, extort an added show of affection—a bit of cupboard love—by teasing him with tidbits and delicacies. You can also become a never-failing delight to small children by supplying them with a steady diet of lollipops. Most people don't go the lollipop route with children. But with dogs, unfortunately, they do.

The urge to provide a great variety of foods for a dog is another example of the prevalence of nonsense, in this case endlessly and ably reinforced by the distributors of pet foods who would rather see your pantry stocked with nine different foods (or labels) than one. You and the manufacturer may be pleasured by variety. Your dog couldn't care less. He likes what he has been trained to eat, and he likes it today, tomorrow, the day after tomorrow, and until time runneth out. Indeed, he generally prefers to have the old familiar again and again, and often he is gravely disappointed in a delighftul delicacy set before him unexpectedly—as anyone knows who has tried to palm off a new food on a settled old dog who is content with what he has been eating for years.

And speaking of advertising: It shouldn't be necessary to remind owners that the ubiquitous advertising campaigns mounted to tell you how to feed your dog are not educational programs. Dog food is big business (did you know that more pet food than baby food is sold in the United States today?) and the multimillion-dollar advertising blitz that supports it clearly influences the way dogs are fed. The programs are skillfully designed for a single purpose—to persuade you to buy a particular product and to buy lots of it. There is, of course, something called "truth in advertising," but insofar as it is either enforced or enforceable, it is intended only to prevent the advertiser from making outrageously and blatantly false claims. It is wholly negative. It does not compel the advertiser to tell you the truth or any part of the truth. It permits him to woo you in any way that proves effective—by singing jingles, exploiting your love for the dog, playing on your fears, encouraging your misconceptions, inventing preposterous needs and urging you to satisfy them, appealing to your generosity, your niggardliness, your snobbishness, and by any other irrelevance that might conceivably persuade you to buy his product.

How else can you account for the fact that a canned

product became one of the most popular foods on the market on the strength of advertising that suggested that an all-meat diet was best for dogs? All nutritionists know that it is not only unwise to feed such a diet but also dangerous. But millions of owners *don't* know that. The advertising appeal worked and sales soared until it was demonstrated in several research projects that dogs fed on such a diet often degenerated so badly they had to be destroyed. Then the manufacturer added other ingredients to make the product more acceptable.

And then there are the supplements. Their distributors spend more millions to convince you that you are neglecting your dog if you merely feed him properly. He also needs (the advertisers assure you) cod liver oil, wheat germ oil, wheat germ meal, and extra vitamin E for his heart. Calcium phosphate tablets supply some critical need that you have foolishly overlooked. The hyphenated products—the ACID-MINERALS and the VITAMIN-AMINOS—are obviously more powerful than the unconnected drugs. There are also dozens of liquids containing mysterious substances that will make your dog's coat lustrous beyond compare. And then, if you will only continue to feed mutiple vitamins by the handful—powders, pills or capsules—you will certainly have a superdog who is superhealthy. This is supernonsense. And if you were foolish enough to stuff him with everything the advertisers tell you is essential, Hector would soon be a supercorpse.

A healthy dog needs a balanced diet. Enough of it. Not too much of it. And nothing else. If for some reason your dog does need a supplement, your veterinarian is the person to tell you what and how much he should have. Not somebody selling pills by mail.

The troublesome, recurrent question is: What is a balanced diet for your dog, and how are you to provide it? There are a multitude of answers, long and short. The long answers involve such formidable difficulties that they can be disposed of here almost instantly. Animal nutrition is a vast complication, and if you want to understand it thoroughly, you can go back to college and get a Ph.D. in the field. You won't. Or, you can study the best of the scores of books on the subject and become your own expert. You won't. If you did, you would still face the task of working out a formula, gathering dozens of ingredients, and concocting your own mixture. You won't. And if you were compulsive enough to do all of that, you would still run the risk of falling into some current faddist fallacy or simply failing to make the perfect food you planned. And I hope that you won't do that.

The short and realistic answers are that you will either continue to feed the dog much as you have in the past—a combination of random table scraps and some sort of dog food, or your own home-prepared meals for the dog, or whatever the custom has been at your house—or you will seek and take the advice of a qualified person who *is* expert in the field and *can* give you reliable information.

In the first case your dog *may* get a reasonably sound, balanced diet. That depends on how much you know about food values and requirements, what kind of eating habits you've encouraged in the dog, how concerned and diligent you are in making sure that the dog is actually getting all of the essentials of a good diet. The do-it-yourself plan usually turns out to be a hit-and-miss method that fails as often as it succeeds. A dog doesn't naturally eat what is good for him. A well-fed dog can be ill fed, and an overfed dog can still be malnourished.

From all of this you will have concluded, I hope, that the simplest, easiest, and most reliable way to find out what a balanced diet is and how to feed it properly is to take your dog and your questions to your veterinarian. Let the veterinarian examine the dog and weigh him, tell him what you are feeding and how much, ask him specific questions about the things that are bothering you, tell him you want his advice on food and feeding, and hear what he tells you. This is the only way I know of to get past the ambiguities of on-the-average generalities and to get specific, usable information about feeding the one dog you are interested in.

If you are feeding a commercial dog food—as most owners now are—your veterinarian will want to know what kind you are using. Not all of them are complete and balanced diets. In your supermarket there is at least half an aisle of different types and brands. Most of them have impressive labels that list the ingredients and offer a reassuring chemical analysis of the contents. But what you read there will not tell you—or anybody else—all that you should know about what is in the package. The list will not tell you how much of any ingredient there is, and the percentage of crude protein, fiber, or fat will not indicate what kinds they are or how much is available in the digestive process. What you read is not nesessarily what your dog gets. But it is part of your veterinarian's business to know which of the foods available in your area are reliably and consistently good. If you ask him, he will tell you. Certainly there is no easier way and, in my opinion, there is no better way to find out.

All things considered—and I like to think that in thirty years in practice I must have considered most of them—I believe that there is nothing better for the healthy old dog than one of the good dry commercial foods or the semimoist foods that look like hamburger. Not all of them are ideal. But the best of them are compounded by expert nutritionists and are produced under accurate control and with rigorous standards. They are not the only acceptable foods, of course, and other veterinarians have other opinions. I speak only for me—and from my own experience both as a veterinarian and an owner who has bred and raised a good many more dogs than I actually needed. I find that the dry foods are best.

I don't recommend canned foods. To begin with, I am myself reluctant to buy canned products which, on the average, are 74 percent water. At current prices, that is an expensive way to provide water. But there are other reasons, too. I find that the content of these cans varies greatly from lot to lot, apparently depending on the availability and price of the raw materials. Worse, I have opened many cans that contained not only an excessive amount of tendons and gristle and other useless junk, but also such debris as matches, wads of hair, and cigarette butts. I have discovered so many surprise packages of this sort that in conscience I've had to advise clients not to feed such products, particularly to pups or to very old and vulnerable dogs.

We have also had a number of cases of food poisoning which we traced to canned foods, and I suspect that most of them were due to careless or faulty canning procedures.

One night an old dog was rushed to my office in the throes of what seemed to me to be food poisoning, and I told the owner so. He rejected the idea out of hand. "No way, Doctor, no way. I've got three dogs. They all had the same food and only this one is sick. And they are all leash dogs, too. No garbage. No poisoned carrion." I was puzzled and a little shaken, but we treated the dog for poisoning and he improved quickly. The next morning the man phoned me. "You were right about that dog you are treating for food poisoning. And I know how it happened. I told you I had three dogs. Well, each of them gets half a can of food in the morning and another half at night. Last night I fed two dogs from one can and gave half of another can to the dog you're treating now. This morning I gave the half that was left over to one of the other dogs, and now, ______ ______ it, *he's* sick. I'll have him in your office in fifteen minutes."

There have been too many incidents like that. If you must use a canned food, at least take the precaution of getting a brand that is government inspected. That narrows the field drastically. Read the labels. As far as I know, only one manufacturer is concerned enough about the safety of your dog to be willing to pay for that inspection.

But that one brand is, I think, available all over the United States.

How are you to determine how much food your old dog should have? You could read the label on the package and feed the quantities suggested by the manufacturer for dogs weighing from thus to so. And that would probably work, for a time at least. Your dog wouldn't starve, you can be sure. And since the manufacturer is in the business of selling dog food—and still more dog food—if you followed his advice, there is an excellent chance that you would have a fat old dog before long.

There is another method that *sounds* better and, if it is properly used, *is* better. It has been determined that an average dog of a certain weight needs a certain number of calories to stay trim, slim, and in good health. The average fifty-pound dog, for example, should have about 1,750 calories per day. You can easily find pound-calorie graphs worked out with a curve that will show you the approximate number of calories your dog should be getting. With a little research and mathematics you can establish the per-pound or per-can calorie value of the standard commercial foods. And if you are industrious enough and knowledgeable enough you can even calculate the calories in the tidbits and table scraps you are providing. If you can apply it accurately and conscientiously, this method *will* work.

But calorie counting has its faults. The first and most obvious one is that it requires more effort than most people are willing to give it. Few owners have the patience or inclination to weigh and measure and calculate. Almost nobody can or does translate an after-dinner plateful of scraps—an inch and a half of fat, the remnants of two baked potatoes and one pie crust with gravy—into calories. And how many doggy bones and treats were there? The bookkeeping becomes ridiculous. And the dog gets fat.

A greater problem is simply that the charts and graphs are made for average dogs. And there is no such thing.

There are breed differences. Clearly an old Terrier who is still busy all day long burns up more calories than an old Hound who prefers to drape himself over the end of the sofa and stay there. Some breeds seem to have inherited a compulsion to eat and grow fat, like most of the Pugs and Cocker Spaniels I encounter. How and where the dog lives makes a difference, too. The thirty-pound dog who spends twenty-four hours a day defending the territorial integrity of your wooded acre is not to be graphed with the thirty-pounder who lives in a small apartment and has a twice-a-day parade around the block. And, as you long ago discovered, Hector himself is insistently individual. He won't average out, and the older he gets the less interested he is in conforming.

But more than any of these things, it is his age that determines how much food a dog needs. A young dog can eat about what he can hold and still not gain weight. For two reasons: because when he is young his digestive system is not as efficient as it will later become, and because he is normally so active that he uses energy as though he had never heard of shortages. That balance of high calorie-intake and large energy-output may continue well into his middle years and as long as it does his weight will remain nearly constant. But the time will come when his digestive apparatus begins to extract more calories from each pound of food. His appetite remains large, his energy consumption declines as he becomes more thoughtful and less active, and the difference between income and expenditure is banked away in fat. And he gets compound interest: as he gets fatter he becomes less active, and as he becomes less active he gets fatter—and so to obesity. And all of this happens on the same amount of food that kept him slim and shapely only two or three years before—on exactly the 1,750 calories that it says, right there in the chart, that a fifty-pound dog should have.

To sum it all up: Hector is an individual—a dog of one particular breed, size, temperament, and age living under his own set of circumstances with his own complex of habits and activities. You can't responsibly determine his food requirements by reading a label on a package or by consulting a thousand-dog-average chart. What *should* you do, then? My suggestion is still what it was a few paragraphs ago. Consult your veterinarian.

When the veterinarian weighs Hector, your problem is not likely to be how to maintain his ideal weight. You will probably find yourself among the sinners who have allowed their old dogs to feed beyond their needs and discover too late that they will have to pay for their sins in one of two ways—by continuing to watch their dogs eat their way to destruction, or by forcing them to peel off the layers of fat that should never have been allowed to accumulate in the first place.

You'll take the second alternative. Not everybody *does,* but if you have come along this far, you surely will. Your veterinarian will tell you what your dog should weigh, and he will tell you how to get him down to that weight. It won't take him long to explain how it is done. There is only one way. You will have to reduce the amount of food you give the dog to less than the amount required to support his present activity. You will have to cut his diet until his body uses the fat that it has stored for the rainy day that never came. It is not an easy way, and it is not a quick way. The fat will come off slowly and the dog will be hungry and unhappy for a time. It will be difficult for him, particularly at the beginning, and it will be more difficult for you. But if you persevere, he will survive—and survive much better and much longer than he will if you fail.

The fatter the dog, the longer the travail. To maintain his weight and his health an old dog often needs no more than half the amount of food he ate when he was younger and more active. If he has continued to eat as much as he did at his peak, to cut back even to the proper maintenance level is a severe restriction. But in order to force him to lose weight you are going to have to reduce his diet to a point somewhere *below* the maintenance level. The reduction should not, however, be more drastic than it has to be to make him begin to shed the excess weight. A small dog should not lose more than a quarter of a pound a week and for a large dog half a pound is enough. You may not have noticed how long it took to put ten pounds of fat on your dog. But you will learn, sadly, how long it takes to get rid of them.

The first question every owner asks when he realizes that every day for six months he is going to have to face a hungry dog is: Isn't there a quicker way? No, there isn't. In my opinion there is no quick *safe* way. There are the same kinds of reducing pills that some people take. And they have the same dangers—or more—and the same side effects when they are fed to dogs. I refuse to prescribe them. Nor do I think it advisable to subject a dog to a "crash" diet to reduce his weight in a hurry. Its only advantage is that it shortens the period of discomfort—for the benefit of the owner. For the dog it is simply cruelty. It weakens him, it often creates dangerous deficiencies, and it is an inexcusable assault on the whole system. I don't choose to run those risks.

The dog won't be in agony the whole time that he is losing weight. True, he'll be hungry. But hunger pangs are not pain even for you, and for him they are even less severe. The first three weeks or so will undoubtedly be miserable for both of you. He'll watch you with the saddest brown eyes you have ever seen. He'll beg and he'll cry. He will stand in front of you and drool until you are willing to lock yourself in the bathroom until bedtime to escape from him. He will nearly persuade you that he is about to die at your feet. But he won't. He will only lose weight.

After the first few weeks the dog's stomach seems to be less urgently insistent, and it then becomes easier to live with him. Until that happens, there are a few ways to at least mitigate his distress and yours. There are prescription diets built to be bulky but shy on calories. Or your veterinarian may be able to tell you how you can whip up a similar deception at home. And while the dog is ravenous, he may be willing to consume large amounts of a harmless filler along with his scant portion of dry dog food. The best and most available of these fillers that I have found is the ever-present summer squash. Boiled and served with a little real food, it often brings a full hour's relief to both dog and master.

The greatest consolation during these trying days, however, must be the thought that in time they will end. The fat *will* disappear, and when the old dog is down at last to an acceptable weight, you can begin to feed him decently and without shame. Decently. Properly. Sensibly. But not what he used to get. Surely you won't make that mistake again.

But you will be able to give him a reasonable amount again, enough to maintain his weight and keep him healthy and enough to make him happy again. Since his stomach will no longer demand the quantities of food it used to take to satisfy his appetite, he'll be grateful for what you give him. And you will be grateful that he is grateful. And both of you will have years longer—actually years longer than you would have had—to enjoy the good feeling.

I remember that away back there I told you that you could learn everything you needed to know about feeding your dog in only fifteen minutes. And I realize that I have detained you longer than that. There are reasons. You must have noticed that I have strong feelings on the subject. You must remember, too, that I seldom have time to tell owners as much as I think they should know about food and about the harm that can be done with it. Here I *had* time—and I was uninterruptable.

I don't apologize for the length of this chapter or for its evangelical tone. It is, I think, the most important section of the book. Much of what is said elsewhere in the book—about kidney ailments and creaking joints and failing eyesight—applies to some old dogs sometimes. But food—proper food and proper feeding—is a matter that affects the life of *every* dog. And especially every old dog.

If you remember only one thing from this book, I hope it will be this: You can show your love for your dog by feeding him. By feeding him wisely. But when you overfeed him, you are not giving him *more* love. You are poisoning him.

X
Q's and A's

When you are in a veterinarian's office, always ask questions. If you don't understand exactly what the veterinarian expects you to do for your dog, it will certainly help both you and the dog if you find out before you try to do it. And even if it turns out that your question really belongs in some other conversation, it will tell the veterinarian where he is failing to communicate and get him started where he can do some good.

The most disturbing clients, I find, are those who have no questions at all. I know that I don't always make myself so unmistakably clear that nothing is left unexplained, and the client who doesn't ask me about *something* I save said worries me. I don't know where he is. When a client does nothing but nod, then I have to ask the questions I think he *should* have asked, and fumble around until I find him. It would be easier for me and more profitable for him if he would ask his own questions.

Here are some questions about old dogs that clients often *do* ask. And some very abbreviated answers. Most of them are more fully answered in the likely places in the text—often in more than one context. If what you read here tells you less than you need to know, the index will help you find the section in which the subject is discussed in more detail. The answers there will still be the same, of course—but more so. And more persuasively more so, perhaps.

Can an old dog learn new tricks?
The oldest question in the bag, and often the first to be asked. Yes, of course he can. The copybook maxim is wrong. Until an old dog is actually in his dotage, he will learn willingly and well. Those performing dogs you see will keep on polishing their tricks and increasing their repertoires as long as they can skip on stage.

Do old dogs become senile?
Depends on what you mean by senile. When they are very old they do become slow and feeble and even quixotic. And certainly their senses are dulled. But they rarely suffer from the kind of confusion and mental deterioration we associate with senility in elderly people.

Will a dog cease to be housebroken when he is old?
Sometimes. When he is very old. But usually not before then.

Do old dogs remember how it felt to be younger?
I don't believe so.

Does an old dog suffer more or less than a young dog in hot weather?
Probably more. His circulatory system is not as good as it was when he was young, and his thermostats don't work as well.

Should an old dog wear a coat in cold weather?
I don't recommend it except in extraordinary circumstances. But obviously it would be wise for a short-haired

old dog to wear one if he were to be exposed for hours in subzero weather. Or in milder weather if he has been sick.

If a dog's muzzle is gray, does that mean he is old?
No. Many young dogs gray prematurely—just as some people do.

Does an old dog become mean and snappish?
Not always, certainly. And not necessarily. Like people, old dogs sometimes become crotchety and irritable. And like people, some do snap.

Is it safe to let a child play with an old dog?
That's an unanswerable question. What child, what dog, what kind of play? Often it *is* safe. But, especially with a big dog and a small child, there is always an element of risk. So the rule has to be: No—not unless an adult is there.

Are old dogs more or less likely to get lost than young dogs?
More—much more. A very old dog can easily become bewildered, wander away from home, and die before he finds his way back.

Can an old dog adjust to a new home?
Usually very well—with the right home, the right people, and the right help in making the adjustment.

Are there retirement homes for dogs?
Not that I know of, unfortunately. Or—judging by the reports of the quality of the care in some retirement homes for people—perhaps fortunately.

Can a well-trained old dog be given more freedom to range?
Not if you love him.

With all the advances in medical knowledge, is the life expectancy of dogs longer today than it was twenty years ago?
On the *average,* yes. More young dogs are living to be old dogs. But there is no evidence that the oldest are living much longer than they used to.

How long can a well-trained old dog continue to compete with a well-trained young dog?
It depends on the tasks, but for a long time if the competition doesn't involve extraordinary strength and stamina. Some dogs keep on winning obedience contests as long as they are able to jump. I once saw a twelve-year-old Gordon Setter win a field trial in which every other dog was less than four years old. And his performance was a thing of beauty.

Are there dog cemeteries?
Of course there are. I know of many. And so does your veterinarian.

How often should an old dog be examined by a veterinarian?
Once a year at least. And more often if he is very old or has chronic problems.

What kind of dogs do veterinarians have?
The veterinarians I know have all sorts of breeds and mixed breeds. The only common denominator that I have been able to find is that they are always gentle dogs.

Do dogs have diseases that can be transmitted to human beings?
Yes. People usually think only of such things as rabies and ringworm. But there are many common bacterial diseases that affect both dogs and man. There are also a number of

very rare diseases that occasionally are passed from man to a lower animal or the other way around.

Should an old dog have a diet of varied foods?
He doesn't want, need, or expect a varied menu. Even if he did, most commercial foods have *twenty-five* or more ingredients—each of which he recognizes by smell. Enough already.

How much weight—beyond his normal, mature weight—should a dog be allowed to gain as he grows older?
None.

Is it safe to switch an old dog from one type of food to another—from canned food to dried food, for example?
Yes. Not only safe, but sometimes advisable. But if possible it should be done gradually both to prevent digestive disturbances and to avoid distressing the old boy.

How much meat should an old dog have?
He doesn't *have* to have any. He does need protein, either animal protein or vegetable protein. That he will get in any sound, balanced diet—which is more than a short-answer subject. See the chapter on food.

Is fat in his diet bad for an old dog?
No. On the contrary, a reasonable amount of fat is good for a healthy old dog. And if his digestive system will tolerate it, a bit of extra fat from time to time may help to keep his coat sleek and shiny.

Now that he is older my dog eats much less, but he still remains healthy and in good flesh. Why?
Because an old dog's digestive system is more efficient than it was when he was young. Because he doesn't squander energy the way he used to—and therefore needs less fuel.

And because he's one of those rare old dogs who doesn't have a compulsion to eat more than he needs to.

My dog is lazy and he gets fat because he doesn't exercise. What can I do?
Your dog is fat because you feed him enough for a dog who does get exercise. Feed less. And read the chapter on food.

Do dogs get fat because of glandular disturbances?
Perhaps one in fifty thousand.

Do old dogs need extra vitamins and supplements?
Some do. Most don't. A great many of the Methuselahs I have known were never given vitamins or minerals. If your veterinarian thinks that supplements might help your dog, he will suggest that you try feeding them for a month. If the dog looks better or acts better after he's had them, that's excellent evidence that he needed them.

Will an old dog eat enough to make himself sick?
Some will. If your old dog is a glutton and he has been on a restricted diet for a while, he might well overeat to the point of sickness—if you gave him the chance.

Are there special prescription diets for dogs?
Yes, there are. For a number of common conditions. They are convenient, and some are very helpful.

Are sweets bad for an old dog?
I have never found that they were.

Is milk good for an old dog?
Certainly. It's an excellent food. And no matter what the old wives tell you, it does not cause worms. Skimmed milk is mildly laxative.

The pupils of my dog's eyes seem to be turning gray. Why?
Not the *pupils.* They are the expanding and contracting *openings* which regulate the amount of light entering the eye. If it is a general graying of the *lens* that you see, it is an indication of hardening of the arteries, lenticular sclerosis.

Is the degree of graying in a dog's eyes a reliable indicator of his age?
Not really. Hardening of the arteries is, of course, often associated with aging. But sclerosis does not begin at any predictable age, it varies in severity from dog to dog, and it progresses at different rates. The amount of gray in a dog's eyes is at best an uncertain indication of an approximate age.

Does an old dog with cataracts always go blind?
No. A cataract is an opacity, a whitening, of part or all of the lens. As the area grows and becomes more opaque, the light passing through the lens is cut down and the vision reduced in proportion. Some cataracts never become so dense that they exclude all light. Cataracts sometimes develop in only one eye and when they do appear in both, they often develop at different rates.

Do dogs get glaucoma?
They can. See the section on eye problems.

How can I test my dog's eyesight?
It's difficult to actually *test* his sight. You can't use an eye chart. If the dog gets around easily even in subdued light, he sees well enough. You probably won't know that his sight is impaired until he begins to bump into things.

Are dogs color blind?
Yes. They see only in shades of gray, as in a black-and-

white photograph. Presumably, with a dog a dark green registers as dark gray, and an orange-red appears as a light gray.

Do old dogs get cavities in their teeth?
Cavities are rare in dogs, old or young. Caries are the least of their problems.

Do old dogs lose their teeth?
Some do, some don't. Many old dogs keep a fine set of teeth to the very end. Some begin to lose teeth at middle age. *When* they lose them seems to be determined by genetics more than anything else.

If an old dog gets an infected tooth, should it be extracted?
Of course. One bad tooth makes two more, and so on to big trouble. Besides, the toxins and bacteria may spread through the system and cause many other difficulties.

Does chewing bones help or harm an old dog's teeth?
Gnawing a big, hard bone occasionally won't harm the teeth, certainly. And it may be of some help in preventing the buildup of tartar. But a bone that the dog can splinter is a danger.

Can an old dog be operated on?
Yes, unless he is actually feeble or has some condition that makes surgery impossible. Age alone does not preclude it. In fact, I have found that old dogs tolerate some forms of anesthesia better than young dogs.

Should an old dog still get distemper inoculations?
Indeed he must. It is true that some old dogs do develop a surprising immunity to distemper. But others never do. There is no practical way to tell about your dog, so you *must* have him inoculated.

Do old dogs ever recover from a stroke?
Often. Much more frequently than human beings do.

Do all old dogs cough and wheeze?
No. Many do—but the wheezing is a symptom of a disease condition and not merely a sign of old age.

What causes arthritis?
Arthritis is a term used to describe scores of different conditions that appear to be related. But what causes it (or them)—either in people or dogs—is still unknown.

What is jaundice? How serious is it?
Jaundice is a symptom, not a disease. It is the result of an excess of bile which causes the skin and various membranes to take on a yellow or yellowish-green color. There are many possible causes, many of them associated with liver disorders. It is a sign of danger and it should never be ignored.

Just recently the hair on my old dog's forefeet has turned rusty red. Why?
Bacteria from gum infections mixes with saliva, which sometimes moistens the dog's forefeet while he is resting. When the saliva dries, it creates an odor which causes the dog to lick his feet. This adds more saliva, which gradually stains the hair that reddish color.

What causes convulsions?
There are many possible causes—diseases affecting the brain (of which epilepsy is the most common), low blood sugar, toxins resulting from kidney failure, internal parasites, poisons, injuries, to name a few of the most likely ones.

What is normal temperature for an old dog?
The figure is not quite as precise as it is for people. The

average normal temperature is 101° F. It is generally a bit lower early in the morning and somewhat higher in the evening.

Can I keep an outdoor dog in the house after he gets old?
You can, and sometimes you should. He may need to be protected from weather extremes. And if you take the time to housebreak the old hunter properly, both of you will enjoy the change.

Can I ship my old dog by air safely?
I assume that this is something that you have to do, not something you plan to do because it is quick and convenient. If you *must* ship him by air, you can—provided he is in good physical shape and is still emotionally supple and adaptable. If you are doubtful about his condition, you would do well to consult your veterinarian. A sedative or a tranquilizer is sometimes indicated. And he should, of course, be picked up at the airport as soon as he arrives.

Is there a Blue Cross kind of insurance program for dogs?
Plans of this sort have been tried a number of times. As far as I know the only going one operates in a limited area in California. Still, it does sound like an idea that should be developed further.

Is it safe to give cortisone to an old dog?
For a veterinarian to prescribe it? Yes. There is a calculated risk involved in all medication, and the veterinarian must weigh the possible risks against the potential benefits every time he prescribes any drug. Cortisone is one of the steroids which can be of great help in some conditions in old dogs.

Should I add anything to the dry commercial food I am giving my old dog?
Not necessarily. As long as he is in good shape, he'll prob-

ably continue to thrive on it just as it is. If he has problems, your veterinarian may suggest additives of some sort. But there is no reason for you to try to beef up the food just because you have a vague feeling that it might be good for the old boy.

If a dog drags his bottom along the ground, does that mean he has worms?
It might or might not mean that. The same reaction is often caused by an accumulation of secretions in the anal glands. Or it could be caused by a persistent itch of any kind at the base of the tail or around the anal area.

Does an old dog naturally become constipated?
No. Nor does any other dog. Constipation is *un*natural.

What causes a dog to have bad breath?
Any one of several conditions. Occasionally it is caused by constipation. Sometimes by an infection in the fold of the lower lip. But the most frequent cause, I think, is an infection of the gums.

My dog doesn't chew his food. Is that bad?
Only insofar as it offends you. There are nibblers and gobblers. And fortunately dogs' stomachs are designed to handle chunks of food—chunks so large that you are astonished that he can even get them down.

Can anything be done about flatulence in an old dog?
Yes—though it is difficult to eliminate the problem entirely. In some cases, at least, flatulence is probably caused by a lush growth of intestinal flora. Diet is generally a factor. An excessive amount of protein—meat most commonly—is likely to be one of the causes, and changing the diet to reduce the protein content often brings considerable improvement. Charcoal dog biscuits are not a cure, but they are sometimes very helpful.

Do old dogs have allergies?
Yes. But there are no short answers to questions about allergies. The problem is discussed at some length elsewhere in the book.

We're giving up our house and moving to an apartment. Can our old dog make the adjustment?
If you can, he can. But both of you may need some help. For ways to help him, see "When He's Very Old" and other relevant sections.

How long will old Penelope go through her seasonal attractiveness for males?
Usually for ten or eleven years. After that she begins to skip heat periods and those that do occur are generally so slight that they pass unnoticed—by you and the neighbor's dog. But *don't*—repeat—don't take chances because Penelope has just celebrated her tenth birthday.

When will old Hector stop paying attention to the opposite sex?
You'll have to wait to find out. About 50 percent of the old dogs begin to be disinterested after they are eleven or twelve years old. The other 50 percent lose interest when they cease to breathe.

Can dogs be neutered after they are old?
Yes. But it is generally not done unless there is a compelling reason. It *is* done if it is necessary to remove a tumor or treat an infection, and it is usually successful.

Are there "gay" dogs?
I doubt it. Hermaphrodites do appear from time to time, but they are anomalies. Hormonal imbalances caused by tumors and infections of the testicles or ovaries often cause changes in secondary sex characteristics. But the masculine-looking and -acting female generally seems to have normal

reproductive instincts. And many males with feminine mannerisms and underdeveloped testicles have the usual sexual interest but simply don't try hard enough to effect a mating.

Are there contraceptive pills for dogs?
Yes. They have been used successfully in Great Britain and Europe for a number of years, and they have now been approved and released for use in the United States.

Are there intrauterine devices for dogs?
Yes, but—

Until what age can a bitch have pups?
I once attended an eleven-year-old who was having her first litter—and it was not a happy event. I have heard of bitches twelve years old having puppies. And that is not recommended either.

What should I do if an old bitch is accidentally bred?
Get her to the veterinarian on time—within a day, or two days at the most.

How can I keep a spayed bitch from becoming fat?
The same way you keep an unspayed bitch from becoming fat—by feeding her the proper amount of food.

Can anything be done about incontinence in an old dog?
In 95 percent of the cases an occasional pill will eliminate the problem.

XI
When the End Comes

The loss of an old dog, even the fear of losing him, is no small matter. Ever. Or for anybody.

It is a special sorrow. Of all pets the dog most diligently entrenches himself in the hearts and habits of everybody in the household. However conscious his owners are of the gulf that separates him from humans, once a dog is installed in a family, he almost inevitably becomes an active and participating member. He waits for no invitation. He is marvelously adept at insinuating himself into the routine of a home. And almost always he is encouraged to share in the activities around him. He is trained and cajoled and enticed to participate, and the more eagerly and joyously he responds, the more he is valued. And so a kind of associate membership is created for him and he fills his special place abundantly.

But adaptable and resilient as he is—and living with man he has had to make remarkable adjustments throughout his history—he cannot alter the biological limitations of his life. He ages by his own calendar, still basically the same as the one that limited the lives of his canine ancestors. No matter how different his present circumstances are, he grows to maturity, lives and dies on a schedule established eons ago. Biologically he soon becomes the oldest member of the family. It is he who first experiences the pangs and discomforts of old age, and by the time the children who played with him in his puppyhood are entering adolescence, he is approaching senility. And so it often happens that when it comes, his death is the first to touch close to the family.

Even though the old boy may have lived his full allotted years, and even though the end may have been predictably near for some time, there is inevitably a sense of loss and bereavement in the family when he dies. And though there is often a show of dry-eyed fortitude and gruff manliness, the pain can rarely be concealed.

I see no reason why it should be. The owner knows full well that a dog is a dog and that however lovable and cherished he was his death is not to be equated with the loss of a human life. But that doesn't mean that it must be accepted unfeelingly. Only a woefully insensitive person could fail to feel some grief, and only a resolutely restrained and private one could fail to show it. I am unable to understand why some people seem to feel that to cry a little when old Hector goes is an embarrassing sign of weakness. I think that tears are a natural response and I somehow feel uncomfortable with a person who can say good-bye to an old dog with a perfunctory pat on the head and a stiff upper lip.

Most owners are, of course, deeply and visibly disturbed when they must be told that there is nothing more that can—or should—be done to prolong the life of their old dog. For some it is an extremely difficult moment—as it is for the veterinarian. I have tried endlessly to find ways to ease the impact. And I still do. But there simply is no painless way to make the announcement. However gently it is put, it still hurts.

Nor is there any way to predict the owner's reaction. Often I am impressed by the grace and resignation with which some people are able to accept the fact. Occasionally I have been astonished by people who, through their tears, have been moved to reach out to console *me*—a kind of apology, it seems, for having involved me in their private sorrow. Less often—but still not infrequently—a distraught owner will lash out at me for having permitted him to lavish so much love on an animal when I must have known that it would end in sorrow. And always there are those who show every sign of gratitude for the veterinarian's concern during the old dog's last illness and for his help, perhaps, in selecting a new dog for the family—and then never again return to his office, presumably because of the painful associations with the death of the first dog.

In most homes the family dog is a house-connected responsibility, and even in these days of conscious and self-conscious liberation, his routine health care is left largely in the hands of the woman of the house. His trips to the veterinarian, like the children's excursions to dancing school and to the orthodontist, are supervised by Mother. Hector's checkup appointment is arranged, if possible, either early on the return trip from the station or after the nursery-school pickup in the afternoon. The name, Mrs. Clarissa Smythe, on the owner's card does not mean that the lady is a widow. It says only that she is the medical officer in the family. It is common for the veterinarian to see Mr. Smythe only in connection with a weekend emergency. And when the dog is a terminal case.

If a man suspects that the old dog has reached the point of no return, he is likely to bring him to the veterinarian himself. Masculine protectiveness is expected (or demanded) in our society, and he feels an obligation to spare his wife the pain of hearing the veterinarian say that the end has indeed come. The impulse is a laudable one, I suppose, but it is the sort of kindness that usually doesn't work altogether for good.

It is generally less difficult, I think, when spouses

choose to face the hard moment together. The person who comes alone is often faced with the necessity of making a jarring decision on his own—a burden which, understandably, he would rather not assume even though he has his spouse's permission (if that is the word) to do what he thinks is best. Worse, it then becomes his duty to carry the news home to the other for what can sometimes become a long and painful recapitulation.

Though I have been accused (by my own offspring) of an antiquated kind of shoulder-to-shoulderism and a share-the-pain philosophy, my experience with hundreds of these unhappy interviews convinces me that there is indeed some comfort in sharing. When both people are present, the veterinarian at least has the opportunity to discuss the facts at first hand, to answer questions, and to help resolve whatever doubts may exist. It is part of your veterinarian's job to advise his clients as well as to treat their dogs, and there is no sensible reason to limit the help he can give you to a single member of the family. There is in everyone, I think, a natural impulse to support and sustain a companion in pain, and to be able to accept help is often as important as giving it.

Parents are always concerned about how seriously the dog's death will affect their children, and often in their anxiety they magnify the problem unnecessarily. Their reasoning seems to be that if they, as mature adults, feel the loss deeply, then the children, who are far more vulnerable, are likely to be dangerously disturbed. They fear that the death of the dog—who has often been a lifelong playmate—will leave such a void in the child's life that he will face a long and difficult period of adjustment. It seems reasonable to expect some such reaction—and like many well-anticipated difficulties, it seldom occurs.

The death of the dog does, of course, disturb a child, particularly if it comes without warning. But it has been my experience that the parents' fears are almost always worse than the reality. Either the parental anxieties are exaggerated or the children are generally more capably resilient than we think they are. Whatever the reason, the period of grief and bereavement is likely to be far shorter than expected. Many parents have told me with lingering disbelief that what they had feared would be an excruciating crisis turned out to be almost anticlimactic and that a relatively brief burst of tears and outward sorrow was quickly followed by a surprisingly easy acceptance of the loss. Few parents have ever reported any prolonged difficulties. Occasionally a child will miss a day or two of school or his parents will be conscious of signs of withdrawal and a sagging of interest in his usual activities. More often the reaction is even less evident, sometimes so casual that I have known sensitive parents to worry for weeks about a possible delayed response—until, in fact, they had been repeatedly reassured by the child's own easy willingness to talk about the dog's death.

Nevertheless, parents will, of course, offer the child as much help and comfort as the child needs and will accept—without thrusting it upon him. There is no sensible way to advise a parent how to do that, but as far as I can see, the most obvious ways are still the most effective. It is important, I think, that the parents make themselves as freely available to the child as they can, not to hover over him and console him, but simply to be there when he needs them. And it helps, too, if they make some special efforts to plan programs which make it possible for them to participate in activities which the child particularly enjoys. At times like this a good schedule is a full one. And as all parents know, the uses of distraction are many. The chief danger, it seems to me, is that some parents tend to magnify the problem and often continue to discuss it too anxiously after the child is well along in the sequence of forgetting and healing.

In my opinion, the one serious mistake that parents are likely to make is to try to conceal the fact that the dog has died. And that, I think, is both a useless and inexcusable deceit. Not only does it fail to protect the child from an unhappy experience, but also it almost always ends in damaging the child's trust and confidence in his parents. However well intended, it is a bad idea that does nobody good. Parents today are less willing (I hope) than they once were to practice deception with their children. At any rate, few of them ask me to participate in such schemes. And when they do, I flatly refuse.

I have already made my mistakes. I remember only too well agreeing to take part in one such intrigue in the early days of my practice. A man and a woman once brought in an old dog who was in great pain and far beyond the help of any treatment. When I told them that it would be a kindness to relieve him of his suffering, they readily agreed—but only on condition that I help them conceal what had happened from the children. And foolishly I accepted the deal. While the dog was being hidden away in the kennels, the parents coached me on the details of the story they had concocted, and when the children (three subteen-agers) were brought in, I lied to them solemnly. Their parents and I had decided, I told them, that old Ted was very sick and that the only thing that we could do for him was to send him off to a great farm that I knew about—a place away up in Vermont where he could run free in the fields and woods and where (vaguely and indefinitely in the future) he might get well.

It was a dirty little job, and I am ashamed to say that I did it well. But there was more to be done, for the parents either chose to continue the charade or were unable to extricate themselves from the proliferating consequences. Every few months for the next two years those children called me to ask how old Ted was getting along, and I was forced to manufacture plausible but carefully inconclusive reports. Inevitably there came the day when the eldest—by then a delightful teen-aged girl—called in high anticipation to tell me that the family was planning a trip through New England—and that they would at last have a chance to see old Ted again. Where was the farm and how could they find it?

Totally unprepared for that, I stumbled all over the telephone until I could contrive another lie: I didn't have the address in mind, it was inconvenient to look for it at the moment, but I would try to find it, I surely would, and when (if) I found it, I would call her. So I didn't look, I didn't find it, and I didn't call. But she called me. And I crawled still further into trouble by inventing a preposterous story about a lost address book and my desperate search for it.

Enmeshed in the thing so deeply that I couldn't even hope to escape exposure, I shifted nimbly to indignation and in no time at all was able to work up a severe case of injured innocence. From a strong new position of moral rectitude I was able to call the girl's father and tell him plainly that I thought he had done a wicked thing, that I deeply resented being made a part of this unforgivable deception, that honesty was always the best policy, and that unless he was prepared to tell the children the truth at once, I would be forced to do it for him. I suppose that the poor man was somewhat stunned—or amused—to be lectured so vehemently by a singed sinner who had so recently been his willing coconspirator. At any rate, he quietly agreed to set matters straight. And I subsided.

This is, of course, another of those unfinished stories, for naturally I never heard from the man or his family again. I have sometimes wondered if the man actually did make full confession to the kids. And if he did, whether he called them all together and told them the truth, or chose instead to let the fraud seep out gradually—which might have been easier and worse. And I wonder how the children reacted when they discovered that their parents (and I) had been "protecting" them all that time. It's a pity I don't know the end. It's the kind of story that deserves a memorable moral. Perhaps something like: You can fool all of the people some of the time . . .

Tell the children the truth. With as much gentleness and compassion as you can manage. But tell them the truth.

They will survive, and they will not be scarred for life. There are child psychologists—and a growing number of them, I believe—who are convinced that an experience of this kind may in the long run be beneficial for a child. In the past, when the family was commonly part of a larger clan group, a child was early initiated into the natural cyclic aspects of life. Births were marked with parties where throngs gathered to celebrate, and deaths were solemnized with funeral rites that, by modern standards, were prolonged and often agonizing. But today children often grow to maturity—and even to middle age—with only a distant knowledge of death, without having experienced the loss of anyone they loved or even knew. For such people the death of one who is very close can be a calamitous blow for which they are in no way prepared. It seems reasonable to think that some earlier familiarity with death—even the death of the family dog—is an experience that can to some degree reduce the crushing impact of the first encounter with death close at hand.

Parents who show great concern for children in these circumstances sometimes forget that others in the house may feel the loss more deeply—the old people in the family. And often their distress *is* deeper and more abiding. The common assumption is that the aged, who have seen much of life and death, are unlikely to be disturbed by the loss of an animal. It is undoubtedly true that some individuals, as they grow old and slip into senility, focus their concern more and more exclusively on their own survival. But there are far more, I think, who become increasingly dependent on attention and a show of affection, and it is common for such people to develop a profound attachment to a dog who responds so willingly and completely. For them the loss of the dog can sometimes be a jarring blow.

Grandmothers are no longer fragile, porcelain shelf

figures, and surely everybody knows many peppery old ladies who are actively destroying stereotypes and living a second or third life with great verve and enthusiasm. But not all old people are activists brimming with vivacity, and even those who seem to be resolutely independent are not always as protectively insulated as they would have you believe. It may well be that they have in the past survived misfortunes with remarkable fortitude. But there comes a time when even the sturdiest person may at last feel that the pummeling has become intolerable, and some unfortunate event—even a relatively minor one—can trigger an alarmingly disproportionate response.

That sometimes happens when the old dog is snatched away—most often, I think, with a person who has not yet had sufficient time to recover from recent sorrow or despair. Typically, the reaction takes the form of a mild melancholy which passes with time and the help of other members of the family. But if it occurs at a time when it seems to be the culmination of a series of misfortunes—illness, for example, or the news of the death of an old friend—there is the chance that sadness may grow into sorrow, and that sorrow may become deep melancholy.

With problems of this kind, prevention (as always) is far better than cure. Generally, I think, it is a time for doing and not for talking. It may be that the time is right to revive the plans for a long-delayed visit to a friend or to a member of the family a city or two away. Or just a plain vacation if the season is good. Or, if that seems too demanding, perhaps a few days of desultory shopping.

And though we've used a grandmother example here, it might well have been more perceptive and more to the point to remind you that the lorn grandfather is equally subject to depression. He too has his glooms, and if there are signs that he is off stride, it may be prudent to consider the tonic benefits of a trip or a new and challenging garden project.

Old people living with their families are generally

not seriously disturbed, but old couples and those living alone are sometimes deeply bereaved by the loss of an old dog they have had for many years. Theirs is a special case. As they grow older and their outside interests and activities are increasingly restricted, the companionship of the dog becomes a comfort and a support. And as the dog grows older and more crochety, they provide for him with growing attention. If his appetite lags, food is specially prepared to tempt him. In inclement weather he is carefully bundled up before being taken on walks—walks which are necessarily more frequent for him and which, accomplished at a staid pace agreeable to the leader and the led, are therapeutic for both. For the owners the dog is a happy tie to a more active past and a welcome responsibility for the present.

Old people who for years have lived alone with a dog often become intensely preoccupied with his care and welfare. He is their last bulwark against solitude, one of the few dependable comforts and solaces in a dwindling life. Sometimes, indeed, the responsibility for the care of the dog becomes a critical factor in supporting the owner's own will to live. Everybody has known frail old couples who managed to survive many long, unlikely years, each of them seemingly motivated by the fierce desire to sustain the other. And any veterinarian can tell you of cases in which the lives of a lonely owner and his or her dog were similarly entwined. I have known several.

Sometimes the fear of *not* surviving the dog is almost as great as the fear of losing him. An owner who can summon up the fortitude to bear the prospect of the dog's death may not be able to abide the thought of leaving his dog homeless. Where in the world, he asks, is there a place for a tired old dog without an owner? Where, indeed. So every year hundreds of people provide for surviving dogs in their wills, either leaving funds to the animal himself or settling a sum on a person who agrees to provide care for the rest of the dog's life.

For some people even the formal provision of an annuity is too uncertain. Some years ago an old dog was brought to me for euthanasia. I knew the dog well for I had been seeing him for more than ten years. But this time he was not with his mistress. She had died that morning. The person who came with him, a friend of the owner, brought cash (how carefully it was planned) and written instructions from the owner that the dog was to be destroyed and buried with her. For months I had been keeping the dog alive and relatively pain-free only because of his owner's entreaties, and I was willing enough to put him to sleep at last. But I warned the person charged with this last duty that I had been told that it was illegal to have an animal buried in a grave with a human body. Nevertheless, the messenger felt honor-bound to follow instructions and took the dog's body away. Later he told me—with the sense of having faithfully discharged a risky obligation—that with the connivance of the gravediggers he had been able to place the dog on his mistress's coffin and to stand by to see that it remained there when the grave was covered. To such lengths will lonely people go.

Certainly I don't mean to suggest that all old people are likely to be inconsolably stricken with grief at the loss of a dog. But some *are* profoundly disturbed. They are bereft, and they often grieve alone. The veterinarian who knows such a person, and thinks that he may fail—or refuse—to tell others of his loss, will often spend much time trying to locate one of the owner's friends. Someone should be told what has happened. And he should be warned that for a lonely old person the death of his dog may be as crushing as the death of an old friend. Which is what it is. It should be treated with the same cautious concern.

These are good times for dogs, and particularly for old dogs. More than ever before people are willing to make the effort to take care of their dogs sensibly, and veterinary medicine—though it still has far to go—has made it possible to keep them active, comfortable, and pain-free almost to the very end.

But there is a price for these benefits. The longer the dog lives—the more successful we are in protecting him from the debilitating diseases of old age—the more likely it is that the day will come when you will have to decide when his life must end. You try not to think of that possibility. You hope that mercifully the dog will die peacefully and quietly in his sleep. And sometimes it happens that way. But when it doesn't, when the dog at last goes into a slow decline from which there is no relief, it will be up to you to decide when his life has become only a burden from which he should be released. It is a difficult decision and a painful one. When the time comes to make it, you will need help.

You will need help because, in the first place, you are not qualified to judge the dog's condition. It is true that you know your dog better than anyone else. And nobody doubts your ability to see. But to understand what you see is something else. Even an experienced veterinarian often finds it difficult to evaluate a situation properly. Symptoms are seldom totally clear, and they are not always what they seem. A condition that appears disastrous to you may be far less serious than you think. And there is, of course, an obverse to the coin. The fact that a dog is not whining or prostrated cannot be taken as proof that he is not in serious pain. I have known many gentle and kindly people who have mistakenly permitted their dogs to suffer long, intolerable pain simply because they were waiting patiently for signs the animals would never be able to give them.

And you will need help because you and your family will face psychological difficulties which, though they are less than overwhelming, are more than trivial emotional incidents. Much of this book is concerned in one way or another with your attachment to the old dog, and it would be foolish to suggest here that the decision to end it could be less than painfully difficult. You could—and many people do—choose to confront the situation stoically and alone. And you would not find the experience unbearable. But I see no virtue in courting unnecessary pain. I think it is only sensible to seek and accept whatever help is available. If discussing the problem with a knowledgeable person will make it easier—and I believe it will—you should do that.

Nobody is better prepared to provide the facts and the perspective you need than your veterinarian. He knows, as you can't, how serious your dog's difficulties are, and within reasonable limitations, he can chart the changes you may expect. If he believes that there are still effective ways to strengthen the dog or alleviate his pains, he will tell you—what they are, how well and how long he thinks they will work, how bothersome or painful they may be for the dog, whether they involve frequent visits to the office or whether you can manage the treatments yourself.

And if he must, he will tell you that there is nothing further that he can do. If he must. To tell a still-hopeful owner that the old dog has at last come to the end of his time is surely the most painful duty a veterinarian has. I know. I have had to do it many times. And it never gets easier.

By asking his advice, you are asking the veterinarian to help you make the decision. You are also asking him to share the responsibility. That is right and proper, and he has an obligation to do that. But you must also remember that it is *your* dog and *your* dog's life, and in the last analysis you must accept the responsibility for the decision.

Don't, please, come to the veterinarian's office with the intention of washing your conscience clean and leaving your dog and his difficulties in his hands. He will be quick to resent any attempt to make him shoulder the whole burden. He has been through that before. And more people than you would expect, after they have been told that the old dog is in intolerable pain and that they must either provide effective relief for him or have him put out of his misery—more people than you would think are capable of staring out of the window and saying, "Well, whatever you think, Doc."

Whatever *you* think. Which, being translated, simply means that the owner doesn't have enough interest or concern or compassion to give the dog the care and attention that he needs. It is worse than that. It means that the owner is trying to force the veterinarian to make a choice: either he will let the dog continue to suffer with an owner who has no interest in treating him properly, or he, himself, must be responsible for ending the life of a dog who might have been saved. In such circumstances many a good and gentle veterinarian has been compelled against his will to keep a dog from months of misery by ending his suffering once and for all. This *you*-decide attitude is a mean evasion of responsibility. It's a dirty little trick that should be unthinkable to any owner.

So don't try to *use* your veterinarian. Consult him. Listen to what he has to say. If there are alternatives, discuss them with him and express whatever doubts you may have. Ask him questions about any problems that may be troubling you. And then have the strength and character to do what you believe is right.

I mentioned questions. I can understand that an owner who has just had to make a painful decision often wants more than anything else to end the discussion as quickly as possible. And certainly I don't want to prolong these sessions unduly. But I do think that they can be too brief. Many owners, in their haste to escape, are willing to leave the office with lingering qualms and doubts, and I have found that the most useful thing I can do is to get them to talk about these feelings. I encourage them to ask questions. And sometimes, if I'm given the opportunity, I try to answer questions that haven't been asked when I think they should have been. The answers don't, of course, resolve all quandaries. But they do at least give the owner an opportunity to sum up his thoughts and perhaps to get a better insight into his own feelings. And that in itself can be helpful.

Nobody can predict what particular problems may arise when an owner has to make a life-or-death decision about his dog. But some questions are common to every such experience, and for his own comfort and peace of mind, I think every owner should have clear and satisfying answers for them. Cases differ, needs differ, questions differ. But here, by way of examples, are some of the questions that I hope are always freely asked and fully answered.

Is the dog in a hopeless condition?

Only your veterinarian can properly answer that. By *hopeless* he means either that he sees no way to prevent the dog's death or that he is unable to relieve or correct the condition enough to permit the dog to live without intolerable pain or disability. When he can, the veterinarian will give you a clear and unequivocal answer. Nothing can be done to save a dog with a massive, inoperable cancer, and he will have to tell you that. On the other hand, he may be able to assure you that the acute symptoms that seemed so alarming to you merely reflect a condition that can be corrected and that there is an excellent chance that with treatment the dog will recover completely.

The great difficulty is that the answer sometimes is neither *yes* nor *no* but *perhaps*. The course of a disease is not always predictable; the effects of treatment vary; individual animals respond in infinitely varied ways. Often the veterinarian can do no more than tell you what the problem is, what the possible courses of treatment are, and what, in his best judgment, he can reasonably expect to achieve.

This *is* an answer: the dog is not in a hopeless condition. But it is an elusive answer that inevitably leads to further questions.

Does the dog still enjoy living?

You want to keep your dog as long as you can. And you should. But you must realize that the time may come when keeping him alive is selfish and cruel. It is simply an evasion to tell yourself that he doesn't want to die. No animal except man reasons, and it is absurd to imagine that a dog can rationally will to live or die. Like all organisms, he continues until life is somehow extinguished even though the end may be excruciatingly prolonged and painful or merely a senseless, unfeeling survival of the body.

It is inhumane to keep a dog dangling in a twilight existence when he has become so senile and feeble and so removed from the life around him that he can no longer have any joy in it. He has no memory of the past and no thought of the future. He has only the suffering and infirmities of the present.

Beyond that, beyond the clear obligation to be decently humane, there is something else which I think many people feel even though few ever mention it. They have a reverence for life—the life that pervades all things. They also feel that in death, as in life, there is (or should be) a certain inalienable dignity. And to allow a dog to linger on in a mere insensible existence seems to them to be depriving him finally of the dignity that is rightfully his. It is hard to talk about such a feeling without sounding ponderous, but it is a factor in many people's thinking, I am sure. And rightly so, I think.

Is the dog in great pain?

This is perhaps not as simple and obvious as it sounds.

The problem is not that you will fail to recognize the common outward signs of pain. From half a mile away you can instantly distinguish the yawp of delight from the yelp that means the dog has been hurt. And there can never be any doubt in your mind when you find him trembling and crying and unable to stand. You know he is hurting.

But how are you to judge what pain he feels without showing these gross signs? It is a mistake, we have already said, to assume he is not in pain simply because he doesn't moan and whimper. Often—indeed, more often than not—a dog will endure a severe, continual pain without a sound. He is more likely to show it only in the way he walks and stands, the way he holds his head, the way he licks and bites himself. A dog suffering the acute pain of a moving kidney stone, for example, may show no outward sign other than a slightly arched back.

Don't depend on your dog to complain when he is hurting. Far from being as clear and explicit as you might expect, the signs of pain are often subtle. And before you decide that the dog is *not* in pain, you'd do well to ask your veterinarian for his opinion. Even he may not always be sure, but he can read the signs better than you can.

Can the dog be kept reasonably pain-free?

Almost always something can be done to provide temporary relief from acute pain. But to find a feasible way to keep an old dog free from pain day in and day out is another matter. There comes a point when it simply can't be done.

The continued use of pain-killing drugs is not a kindness, I think, if they serve no other purpose than to permit a dying dog to live a few days longer. But if there is a practical and humane way to make it possible for an old dog to continue to live comfortably for a reasonable time, you'll want him to have such treatment. But you must remember that in most such cases you are buying only time and that there is a limit to the price you can ask the dog to pay. What kind of treatments will he have to have? How often? How painful are the treatments themselves? How much will the visits to the veterinarian's office distress the dog?

If you have doubts, perhaps the best way to resolve them is to try the treatments for a while to see how they work out. You will soon know. And if the cost in pain and apprehension turns out to be beyond the dog's strength, you will not ask him to carry on just for your sake.

Can you care for the dog properly?

You feel a deep sense of responsibility for your dog, as you should, and when he is old and sick, the very thought that you might be giving up too soon and too easily distresses you. Your impulse will be to assume that you can and must care for him to the very end. But you must also ask yourself: How long—and how well—*can* you take care of him? It is true that you have an obligation to him, but it is an obligation to take care of him properly, not merely to provide shelter for him.

Attending to a sick old dog is not something you can do when and if. It can be a wearisome, demanding, and frustrating responsibility. However willing you are, it is certainly possible that you do not have the strength, the time, or the place to give him the care and attention that he must have. Should he be left alone? When you have to be away from home, will there be somebody there to take charge? Find out exactly what will be expected of you. Think of your schedule for the next week and ask yourself how you are going to manage what must be done.

Nobody has to remind you that to fail to do what you can and should do is inexcusable. That is not likely to happen. But you should be warned, I think, that to promise to do more than you can accomplish is a regrettable mistake. And it is a mistake that you might easily make.

How will others in the family be affected?

You and the dog are not the only ones involved. You will also have to consider the feelings of others in the family.

Usually there are no problems at all. On the contrary, having people to help often makes it possible to keep a dog that you could not otherwise care for. They are at home when you have to be away, they can take him for walks when you are busy, they can help with the feeding and the medication. A child may well feel that he has been promoted to adult responsibility when he is charged with remembering medicine time, and Grandfather may insist that all those short walks are good for his arthritis. Good. Good all the way around.

But you must remember that it doesn't always work out so happily. There is also the chance that an old person who is inclined to be melancholy will find that an ailing dog is a persistent reminder that life is running out. And little children at the boisterous age may have difficulty in remembering that the dog is sick and insist on roughhousing that the dog can no longer tolerate.

You will have to work for some compromise. To some extent you can persuade Grandfather that his attitude is unnecessarily gloomy and you can surely convince the children that the old dog has to be allowed to rest. You preside as equitably as you can. You try. You hope. But if a crisis atmosphere pervades the house, you do what you must. You cannot batter the family to sustain the dog.

Will keeping the dog be prohibitively expensive?

Nobody wants to talk about what it will cost to keep the old dog alive and comfortable. But for most people cost is a factor, and there is no reason to be ashamed to discuss it with your veterinarian.

He knows that for most owners the question is simply how much they *can* do, not what they want to do. It is true that once in a while every veterinarian encounters a despicable character so heartlessly stingy that he won't spend the few dollars necessary to keep his dog alive and well—and I have had my say about such people elsewhere. But for every tightwad there are a hundred owners who, if necessary, are prepared to skimp and save if money is all that it takes to keep old Hector going.

The cost of medical care, for animals as well as for people, is high—too high. And for old dogs there is no Medicare. There is a limit to what a family can or should spend for the care of a dog, and your veterinarian knows that as well as you do. He will tell you if he thinks that the treatments your dog needs are going to be distressingly expensive. But he doesn't know your circumstances, and if costs are a problem for you, you should tell him.

Don't worry. You can talk about money to your veterinarian. He won't think that you are counting out your love for the old dog in dollars and cents.

Will keeping the dog seriously disrupt your life?

It is not perverse, I think, to suggest that you ask yourself if you love your old dog too much. Perhaps that is an unfortunate way to put it. What I mean to say is that over the years your love may have exceeded the bonds of affection which people normally establish with animals. It happens. And sometimes it results in a dangerously excessive concern for the dog.

The very old and lonely, as we have said before, have a tendency to let their values get out of kilter this way. They drift along until they are out of touch sometimes, and it is not uncommon to read distressing stories of poverty-ridden old souls who for years have fed and fattened their dogs while they themselves were undernourished. Such cases are extreme, of course, and fortunately they are rare. But every veterinarian knows soundly competent people who have allowed their lives to be shamefully circumscribed by an exaggerated sense of responsibility for their aging dogs. They become uncomplaining prisoners. They cannot risk being away from home overnight, they have long since abandoned all thought of vacations, and even when their doctors prudently advise them to winter in the South, they choose to tough it out in New England with the old dog.

I expect that I will be the last person in the world to depreciate the owner's obligation to care for a tired old dog tottering on into senility. But there have been times when I felt it necessary to remind an owner that he had still greater obligations. I think that if the day comes when the duties of caring for the dog begin to seriously disrupt the sensible pattern of your life, if his welfare and security seem to have become more urgently important than your own, then you must seriously consider whether your values have somehow, somewhere gone askew.

I sometimes think we dread the *thought* of death as much as death itself. We avoid the very use of the word, we shy away from "morbid" thoughts, we go to absurd lengths to conceal the unconcealable from ourselves and our children—that death, as much as birth, is part of the immutable cycle of life.

We fear for our pets as we fear for ourselves. Death is fearful. The thought of death is taboo. And to many people the thought that they may sometime have to decide to end a dog's life is so profoundly disturbing that they simply recoil from it. Worse, they distort and magnify it. "But I can't let you *kill* him!" I have often heard people say. "I simply can't *kill!*"

I can't believe that this common distortion reflects a real misconception. More likely, I think, it is a cry for reassurance. Everybody surely knows that euthanasia is not killing, with all its violent connotations. And yet a great many people seem to need to be told that it is not an evil thing. However old and evident the facts are, I am afraid that they not only bear repetition; they require repetition.

The decision you are making is not to *kill* the dog.
You are not choosing whether he should live or die.

> You know that his death is imminent and unavoidable. The decision you must make is whether to let him endure a slow and perhaps agonizingly painful death or to end his suffering quickly and painlessly.
>
> You are not depriving him of a life in which he can find joy or pleasure. That possibility no longer exists. You are releasing him from pain and disabilities which cannot be alleviated or cured.
>
> A dog does not fear death. He *feels,* but he cannot *think.* He is totally incapable of abstract ideas. He lives without ever having the equivalent of your concept of *living,* and he dies without knowing that there is such a thing as death.

Euthanasia is an old word. It is Greek and it means, literally, *an easy death.* The concept itself is ancient, and as it relates to human beings, it has been a matter of controversy throughout the history of mankind. Certainly this is not the place to even consider—much less to try to resolve—the endless philosophic, religious, social, and ethical quandaries which centuries of bitter dispute have left unanswered. I mention them here only because I must—because the arguments for and against human euthanasia unfortunately color the attitudes of many people toward animal euthanasia. You must be able to set aside whatever convictions you have about human euthanasia and remember that here we are talking only about animals.

It must already be unmistakably clear that with animals I believe that euthanasia is acceptable and defensible. For all of the reasons implicit in the discussions earlier in this section. It is not only justifiable, but there are times, I think, when there is no acceptable alternative. At such times it is cruelly inhumane, I believe, to refuse to release an animal from an intolerably difficult existence. And beyond that, I also believe that to spare an animal from prolonged and unnecessary suffering is the greatest gift of kindness that you can offer him.

But having said that, I must add that I fully realize

that knowing all of this does not eliminate the pain an owner inevitably feels. I know that what I have said about euthanasia is sound and reasonable. I also know that after many years in practice I am still constitutionally unable to share such a decision with an owner without also sharing his distress. None of us, fortunately, is merely a reasoning machine.

Thinking that they are acting out of kindness, many people unconscionably delay giving their permission for euthanasia. They find reasons to postpone the decision—because they haven't totally given up hope, because the dog really doesn't seem to them to be in great pain, because they can't accept the thought of being without him. More often, I think, owners delay because they are haunted by thoughts of what happened in the days when sick and injured animals were callously and brutally destroyed. Few people today, surely, can remember a time when it was common to shoot horses or when some shiftless old character down the road could be hired to take the old dog and a shotgun for a walk over the hill. That sort of barbarity ended years ago. And yet I am constantly astonished at the number of intelligent people whose thinking is somehow colored by those horrors of the past.

Today there are several accepted methods of euthanasia and all of them are quick, sure, and totally painless. Everybody knows that, of course, but almost invariably an owner asks to be assured and reassured that it is true. It is. Death comes as quietly and imperceptibly as a great, overpowering wave of sleep. It is a sleep. In the method used by most veterinarians the dog is given an intravenous injection of an overdose of a general anesthetic. In less than half a minute—and usually in no more than ten seconds—the dog is totally unconscious. The heart and the lungs cease to function, and he never wakes. There is no resistance, no sign that the animal is making any effort to fight off the reaction. The muscles loosen, there is a sigh of relaxation, and with the last breath all life is gone.

Often—very often—I have heard people witnessing euthanasia for the first time say, "I wish I could be sure of going so easily."

Owners often ask whether they can or should remain with their dog until the end. But that is something for the owner to decide for himself, I think. Death comes so gently and mercifully that nobody could be repelled by what happens. There are those who feel that it is a matter of honor and decency to stand by the old boy to the very end, and I have often seen them go away greatly relieved and reassured in the certain knowledge that the dog had died peacefully.

I try neither to encourage nor discourage an owner's remaining, but I suspect that I am not altogether successful in maintaining a neutral attitude. My own feeling is that by being present the owner is subjecting himself needlessly to pain. As I have said again and again, the dog does not know that he has come to his final moment. But the owner does. And knowing that, he cannot avoid an acute emotional reaction, a hurt which can in no way benefit the dog.

As you rightly suspect, I myself have always chosen not to be present at the last moment. When my fourteen-year-old mongrel had to be put away not long ago, I arranged to have it done by one of my colleagues at the clinic—and on my day off. I wanted a postmortem done, and I asked that the report be left on my desk the next day. I know that absenting myself did not greatly diminish my sorrow. I still cried when I read the report. But now I can at least remember the old dog as he was in life without the need to erase a mental picture of him in death.

How to dispose of the dog's body is something of a problem today. It was less troublesome when most people lived in homes with more than a patch of ground around them, when building codes were rarities and health regulations were minimal and casually enforced. I well remember an old gentleman I used to visit often when I was a boy. He had a beautiful garden and seemed to spend most of his time tending it. At one end there were several magnificent rose bushes, each marking the grave of a dog he had once owned, and as we walked he often stopped before one or another to tell me about the exploits of the animal buried there. It sounds lugubrious, I know, but I still remember many of those stories—and it *was* a beautiful garden.

Today cremation has become the usual and most convenient way to dispose of the body. Most veterinarians provide such service, and often, when there has been euthanasia, it is included in a single fee. You can also arrange to have the veterinarian return the ashes to you. You must understand, however, that this option will add substantially to the expense since, when that is done, the crematorium must be prepared and operated for a single animal, which is not the general practice.

There are those who still feel that burial is preferable. Some, if they have a suitable spot on their property, choose to have the dog buried where they can easily and conveniently visit the grave. Few people, I think, would question the propriety of this practice, any more than I objected to the memorial grove which my old friend had planted over a long lifetime. There is, however, a danger that the burial may be elaborated into a funeral service which itself can be an unfortunate, grief-laden experience for the family. And there is always the possibility that the nearness of the grave may be a perpetual reminder of the loss of the dog and contribute to an unduly prolonged sorrow.

The fact that they do not themselves own ground does not always prevent an owner from finding a suitable site for old Hector's grave. I once knew a woman who for years enjoyed walking her dog on a trail that led along the edge of a cliff above a lake. One favorite objective for an all-day hike was a remote lookout point on a promontory over the water, and she and the dog were often together there for hours. When the dog died, she sought out the owner, got his permission and—at what seemed to me at the time an excessive cost in effort and money—had the dog's body carried up there for burial. Many years later her son and I walked to the old lookout one day and he pointed to a graceful white pine that stood alone above the windswept laurel. His mother had planted it in memory of the old dog. It was, I thought, one of the handsomest memorials I had ever seen.

At one time, years ago, we used to permit people to bury their animals on a hillside near our veterinary hospital. Many of our clients accepted the offer—so many, in fact, that we later had to withdraw it because the stream of mourners on fair Sundays and holidays became depressingly long. For fifteen years one owner brought flowers on the anniversary of his dog's death, and later (perhaps because he had grown too old to make the trip himself) he had a florist put a wreath on the grave. The flowers no longer are delivered, and I suppose that means the old man has died. That's saddening, but I must admit that I am relieved not to see those flowers freezing in the snow every year on the fourteenth of January.

In many areas today there are cemeteries for animals. Like cemeteries for people, some are well planned and cared for and some are not. A few that I have heard about appear to me to be designed mainly (or solely) to extract extravagant amounts of money from grieving owners. They are huckstered into paying for elaborate funeral services, ornate caskets, and mausoleums at staggering prices. Certainly I can understand that a person will want to see a good old dog decently buried, and I am not one to object if he chooses to honor his memory with a suitable marker. On my own property there is a small headstone at the grave of a great little dog, one who by his excellence in field trials became perhaps the most famous dog of his breed in the country. I am proud of the dog and the stone. But it is an outrageous offense to the memory of a dog, I think, to squander thousands of dollars to build an elegant marble monument for him.

Anyone who has the funds and wants to leave an enduring memorial to a dog he loved can do better than to ornament a cemetery plot. Every veterinary school in the country is in urgent need of money to carry on needed research. There are endless and growing lists of promising projects waiting to be carried out—projects which will not only increase our ability to care for and treat animals, but will also contribute importantly (as they frequently have in the past) to our knowledge of human disease. The schools need help, and they will gratefully accept your support in whatever size or form it is offered—endowments, grants for special projects, or modest gifts in lieu of flowers. How better could you express your love for a dog you have lost?

You may have another opportunity to be a benefactor. It is possible that your veterinarian will ask your permission to perform an autopsy—or, as it is called in veterinary medicine, a necropsy. I hope you will agree. The veterinarian is not making the examination merely to confirm his own diagnosis. He is doing it to broaden and expand the knowledge of everyone working in the field. At the very least you will be helping him to further develop his own skills and to increase his ability to provide effective treatment for the dog he will be examining the next day. And you may well be contributing in some small way to the development of knowledge that will have consequences of far greater importance.

XII
Another Dog . . . ?

Will you get another dog to replace Hector?

Yes, probably. The odds are three to one that you will.

That is an arbitrary figure intended to look more authoritative than it actually is. It is the result, in fact, of a thoroughly casual inspection of the client cards in my office files and a random comparison of what they showed with the experience of a number of colleagues in my area. The figure is not the product of the massive effort of a computer, but it does, I think, reflect the facts with round-figure accuracy. A percentage point or two one day or the other can't make any real difference to you. The question is: Will you get another dog? You probably will. So thinking about getting a *new* dog seems to me to be the proper end to a book about *old* dogs.

And before you get it, I think you should think more about the new dog than most people do.

Going back to the three-to-one odds: In my experience, the decision to get or not to get another dog follows a remarkably consistent and persistent pattern. Half of the people who lose an old dog know immediately—or almost immediately—that they want a replacement. A few of them have already picked a successor—the king is dead, long live the king!—and occasionally they have already introduced the new dog into the house so that there will be no interregnum. (More about that later.) A majority simply assume that there will, of course, be another dog. They have always had a dog. To them a dogless house is not a home, and it never occurs to them to think of trying to get along *without* a dog. Usually, if old Hector has been healthy, lovable, and dependably civilized, they plan to replace him with a young duplicate—same breed, same color, same gender. Usually, though not always. A few hesitate for a week or a month and then do what the others have already done—set about looking for a proper pup—and within a few more weeks all of those people have installed a new dog in the house.

The other 50 percent are equally certain and even more emphatic. "Never again!" they say. "Never." Some have suffered so from the loss of the old dog that they are determined never again to open themselves to a repetition of that emotional upset. Others have loved the old dog so long and so well that the thought of looking for another dog to put in his place is simply repugnant to them—a desecration of a memory they intend to keep unsullied. Cooler, less emotional owners often take stock of their situation and conclude that on balance they would be better off without a dog. Their children may have grown up and left home, or they may be planning to move to an apartment or retirement condominium where a dog might be unhappy or unwelcome, or they merely look forward to a time of reduced responsibilities and the freedom to follow the sun south in winter. And there are always a few owners who, having had bad luck with the old dog, simply breathe a sigh of relief at his passing. "We liked him, of course, but he was trouble from the day we got him," they say. "He was a sickly pup, and—you know better than anyone else, Doctor—for ten years it's been one medical problem after another." Or, "He was a loyal old dog. But he was a worry.

He'd bite anybody he thought was an intruder—the meter reader or the Christmas carolers. I still have a lawsuit pending. No more, thank you." All of those in this second half profess to be glad to be relieved of responsibility. All of them are vehemently, vocally positive that they have had their dog. And what happens? Half of *them* have another dog within six months. They bring him in proudly for a checkup. "This—" they say, brushing him up a little for display, "—this is the greatest dog we've ever had. He's the greatest."

The chances, I say, are three to one that you will have another dog.

Will you have another Hector?

No.

That should be obvious to anyone. But apparently it isn't. Another Hector doesn't exist. No two dogs are exactly alike, not even the indistinguishables that you think you see in the same litter. Always there are minimal, invisible variables of all sorts—temperament, innards, standing in the pecking order—and these differences are often accentuated as the pup grows older. But that is only part of it. Owners make their dogs. And you are not the same person you were when Hector was a pup. Now that your girth is greater, your breath shorter, and your rest periods longer, you are going to be a much less exuberant and energetic owner. You'll train the new dog to fit your present taste and convenience. Since you and the pup and the training are all going to be different, the grown dog will certainly be different too. How could it be otherwise?

And yet, as I've said, there is always the owner who thinks that by starting again with a pup of the same sex and breed he will be able to raise another Hector. That's a pity, for when the dog turns out to be something else, the owner is likely to be disappointed. He may have picked an excellent pup and the pup may have all of the makings of a splendid fellow in his own right. But if the owner is so determined to have a replica of Hector that he will be content with nothing else, he will refuse to recognize the dog's good qualities. And often, by persisting in his efforts to mold the dog to fit his own preconceptions, he will actually ruin what might have been an excellent and responsive dog. I've seen it happen. More than a few times.

When you do get another dog, make up your mind that it *will* be another dog, a different dog. You may well decide that you want a dog of the same type as the old one, with the same general characteristics. That's understandable. Why not, if that's the kind of dog you really like? And there is no reason for not choosing one of the same breed, too, as long as you bear in mind what we have just said about individual differences. But don't, I keep telling bereft owners, don't let the choice be a mere rebound reflex. Somewhere in the infinitely varied world of dogs there just might be one that would fit your needs today even better than another Hector.

As a matter of fact, Hector was probably an accident rather than a choice. That is certainly true if he was a first dog, and, habit being what habit is, it is also likely to be true of at least the early replacements. Typically the first dog just happens. He is commonly part of the nest-building process—a version of the dog you remember from your childhood, a tie to the past and a symbol of stability. Often, indeed, he is a pup brought from home, a bit of love and affection gratefully carried from Mom's kitchen to the new house. Or he is an irresistible ball of fluff that a friend offers at the right time. Or he comes to the baby's first birthday party in Grandfather's overcoat pocket. Or, perhaps, he just sat shivering on your doorstep one morning—and nobody in the house could persuade anybody else in the house to call the dog pound. The first dog is generally a happenstance, not really a chosen dog. It may well be that his successor will be the first dog that you have actually selected for yourself. Pup picking is a pleasant experience. And it's even better if it is done sensibly and purposefully.

You'll get lots of advice—all free, some good, mostly

well intended, generally unreliable or worse. As soon as it is known that you are dogless, you will discover that your neighbors' dogs have all had beautiful litters; your friends will urge you to visit the kennel where they found Thor—just *visit* and see for yourself; breed fanciers will dispute over you at dinner parties; a community service person will call to tell you that the town pound has just advertised a "neediest case" dog—beautiful, just beautiful; and your father-in-law will remind you again that you can do as you please, of course, but in his opinion there never was a dog that could equal the Collie—the old-fashioned Collie, that is. Listen to them. Listen to all of them as politely as you can. And think for yourself.

And the first thing you ought to be thinking about—and this is *my* bit of free advice—is whether you *do* actually want another dog. Or need one. Try (with the kind of pseudo-objectivity we all use in such situations) try to weigh some of the important factors involved in the decision. Do you actually want another dog, or are you trying to comfort yourself after the loss of the old fellow? Have your circumstances changed so that you don't really *need* a dog? Will you actually be happier with a dog than without? Should you wait a while to see how you feel? Do you think your way of life may change during the next five or ten years so that it will be impossible or inconvenient to keep the dog? Has your neighborhood developed so that it is no longer a good place for a dog of the sort you like? Are you still active and free-ranging and weatherproof enough to enjoy (not just endure) the daily jaunts? Will your schedule let you care for him as well as you should? Will his companionship offset the responsibilities and restrictions of your freedom? Can you afford a dog? (Yes, that *can* be a factor.) Do you still have the time—and the patience—it takes to train a dog properly?

This may sound like a questionnaire filled with nattering negativism. I don't intend it to be that. I'm not playing devil's advocate, and in this situation I would be the poorest in the world. But I do urge you to think seriously about pertinent questions of this sort before you make a decision. And if it didn't sound so like an old-fashioned schoolmaster's assignment, I'd ask you to use a pencil, too. It's harder to deceive yourself on paper.

I think that you *should* think before you get another dog. And I hope you will. But if you have gotten this far along in this section, I doubt that you will be deterred by a questionnaire. And if you *do* need a dog, you shouldn't be. You may be one of the countless number of people who are actively and consciously unhappy without a dog. And frankly, I hope you are.

There are an astonishing number of reasons why people need dogs. And the reasons themselves are sometimes astonishing. I remember with some fondness a young couple who years ago brought to the office a free-ranging dispute and a dog named Buckie. There was nothing exceptional about the dog—a Standard Amalgam with a vague kinship with half a dozen breeds and a bustling, inquisitive personality. But the couple was memorable. He was a bulky man, upwards of six feet high, extravagantly muscled, and certainly no less than 250 pounds heavy. He looked as though he had been designed by a truck manufacturer to jockey sixteen-wheel rigs on tough, cross-country hauls. And as it turned out, that was exactly what he did. His wife was suitably matched, not quite as high and far less brawny, but still a monumental woman. They appeared to enjoy—and made no effort to conceal—a voluble hammer-and-tongs relationship that seemed to be always on the verge of becoming a physical catastrophe.

The man had brought the dog in for a checkup and inoculations. And his wife had come along, it seemed, to protest both the wisdom and necessity of the trip and (since she suspected that was already a lost battle) to keep the costs down to a level appropriate for a mongrel. The one thing that they were willing to agree about was that some weeks earlier the man had found the dog at a rest area on Interstate Something-or-Other. The pup had been wet, cold, frightened, and apparently hopelessly lost, so the man tossed him up into the cab to warm up while he had his coffee-and-cake break. The dog stayed for the rest of that trip and others, and having proved his mettle on a couple of transcontinental jaunts, was about to be admitted to full membership as a traveling fellow and constant companion. Naturally, Buckie won the battle in my office that day, and as far as I could tell in the occasional routine visits that followed, he remained entirely unscarred by the brouhaha that went on over his head for years.

But hundreds of thousands of miles later, Buckie came to the end of his road. Fearful but still hopeful, the couple brought him to the hospital. When I had to tell them that he couldn't be saved, the man was shattered. He didn't explode, as I feared he would. He slumped on a chair and sat there absolutely silent and unmoving while the tears rolled down his face and splattered in his lap. His wife, plainly stunned, tried to console him with the only outward signs of affection I had ever seen between them. Half an hour later they left in silence. She was holding her husband's hand.

A month or so later the woman came to the office without an appointment and without a dog. She wanted to talk to me about Joe, she said, and when I protested that that I was not qualified to advise her about people problems, she simply talked on. Nobody could turn off Marie.

She had never heard of anything like it, Marie said. Never in eighteen years of marriage had she seen Joe cry until that day in the office when Buckie had to be put to sleep. That did something terrible to him. He didn't eat right, he lost weight, he slept only half the night, he wasn't half the man he used to be. "I mean," she said, with ominous emphasis on a word that she had evidently chosen after careful research, "I mean he's *un-*

manned." And, apparently doubting that I would realize the full implication of what she was saying, she launched without reticence into an account of the physical feats and pleasures of their life that shocked a young but fairly earthy veterinarian.

While I was still trying to gather my wits sufficiently to extricate myself from the conversation, Marie came to her question. "Doctor, it's going to be Joe's birthday. Should I give him a dog?"

She did. And some weeks later the two of them brought him to the office. This time there was no dispute about how much should be spent on him. And from the familiar sound of the hammer-and-tongs exchanges between the two, I gathered that the dog had been splendidly therapeutic.

But that, of course, was an unusual case.

If you want another dog, need another dog, and can take care of a dog properly, get one. But try not to be overly hasty about it. First, because an instant dog is likely to be an automatic, ill-advised attempt to duplicate the old one. Second, because you have had a dog for so many years that you have forgotten what it is like to be without one. You should find out. Third, you need time to consider your needs and circumstances. And finally, if you take time to make a careful selection, you'll vastly improve your chances of getting what everybody wants and few people find—the ideal dog.

But there are exceptions to even a battered maxim like *make haste slowly*. While I was struggling with this manuscript, I had the pleasure of complaining about the difficulties of writing to an old friend, an editor for a publishing house. He read a little, and then to make me more uncertain, pointed out that my precepts and my practice were sometimes at variance. He reminded me of an incident that I had forgotten. His children had teethed on a beautiful little Smooth Fox Terrier called Duz. (It was that long ago, when "Duz does everything!"

was the most detestable advertising slogan on the air.) One morning he and his kids—who were about six and eight years old then—brought Duz to the office to have me diagnose and mend (as they thought) her persistent sore throat. And we had all planned to go to lunch afterward. But it didn't work out so happily. I had to tell them that Duz had an inoperable cancer, that she was in pain, and that the pain could only get worse. All four of us choked up pretty badly when I suggested that they let me keep her and put her to sleep. They agreed and then wandered over to my back yard to talk and cry and wait until I could get away for lunch. It was a grim affair. But when we came back to the office, we all went out to look at my Beagles, lately augmented by two new litters. Fortunately, the kids found a pup of portable age that they liked, and I was able to convince them to take her home to see if she liked it there. And she did—for years.

"So . . ." said my friend after he had reminded me of what had happened that day, "so you recommend a waiting period after a person loses an old dog?" "Yes," I said, "I do."

There is also the theory, mentioned a little way back, that an easy and sensible way to make the transition from old dog to new is to bring in the replacement before the old dog dies. That, too, seems to me to be a questionable practice. It can hardly be easy. The old dog is more than likely to be jealous, sometimes so much so that he will attack the newcomer viciously. Or he will push the pup around so mercilessly that the owner will forever be settling squabbles between them. Or lord it over him until the pup becomes timid and recessive. Occasionally the roles are reversed. Then the old dog may develop a severe feeling of rejection and go into a sudden decline. In that event he will demand an inordinate amount of reassurance and attention. That, in turn, may make the new dog feel like a neglected, second-class citizen. It can become endlessly complicated, and all in all it seems to me to be a dangerous and difficult situation for all concerned. And yet, many people who have followed that practice find that it works smoothly and painlessly. The editor of this book, for one. He says that his old dogs have always shown a paternal interest in the young ones and seem to take pleasure in helping to train them and in showing them the customs of the house. There are, as I say, exceptions . . . always exceptions. They exist to keep veterinarians from becoming complacent and opinionated.

Speaking of veterinarians: Clients who are looking for the ultimate *good* dog—the kind of person who is convinced that there must be one *best* dog if he could only find out what it is—are forever asking what kinds of dogs veterinarians keep. That, it seems to them, is the key, the real tipoff to the secret. And if there were a *best,* I suppose it would be. But I must tell you, sadly, that veterinarians don't have a secret perfect dog. All kinds of dogs are good for something or somebody. And veterinarians, just like people, have all kinds of dogs. If there is one breed preferred above others by veterinarians, I don't know what it is. You are back to square one.

No book is going to tell you specifically when or where or how to move from square one. Nor, as I say, do I think that solicitous friends or well-meaning advisors, however knowledgeable they are about dogs, can do much more than suggest factors you should consider prudently. You are picking a companion, and that involves establishing a relationship based on feelings and attitudes so subjective that they are difficult to identify, much less to articulate. There is the obvious (and dangerous) analogy to choosing a spouse, but I'll spare you that. All I am saying is that nobody can get deep enough into your skull to tell you what dog you want. And having made that pronouncement, I will immediately point out some important considerations I think you should bear in mind.

Without hesitation I will tell you that in my judgments the most important single quality is personality. And as I arbitrarily define it, personality includes the dog's whole character—the way he looks, acts, responds, walks, runs, plays, barks—the total impression you get when you are with him. It is his temperament, attitude, disposition, nature; it is the sum of his reaction to the environment around him. It is an infinite complexity made up of all sorts of contending and divergent forces. Nevertheless, in a dog with a strong personality it becomes an entity, a clear, dominant trait which you feel instantly and can often express in a single word.

There is no limit to the shadings and nuances of personality, and there is a dictionary full of dominant-trait words commonly used to describe them. Let me pick a few out of a hat just to remind you. How many times have you heard a dog described as—spunky, alert, lazy, patient, reliable, pert, watchful, courageous, lovable, amiable, protective, sassy, solemn, comfortable, decorative, inquisitive, loyal, quick. The words go on and on. And so do the dogs. There are groups of dogs and types and breeds and strains. There are mongrels and crossbreeds of high and low degree. There are general characteristics and they are heightened and accented by the individual personality of each dog. With all this to choose from, you are not just picking a dog. You are selecting a manner, a style, a theme. And if I have been reading the signs correctly over the years, you are saying something about what you think of yourself and the world you've encountered.

Many people—perhaps most—make their overall choice on the basis of breed. There are obvious advantages and somewhat less apparent disadvantages to that. When you buy a purebred pup, you know what he is going to look like when he grows up. He has a traceable pedigree, a long line of respectable ancestors, and unless unaccountably he turns out to be a sport, he'll be like them. And if he is bred to another of his own kind, you know what *their* pups will be like. In general, too, the breeds each have certain typical character and personality traits. You have a good idea of how a Hound is going to act and what his attitude toward life is likely to be. Or what to expect from a Terrier. Or a Toy. Or one of the giant breeds. It should be said, however, that these characteristics are not as invariable and absolute as you may think. Within a breed there are often strains with noticeable differences. And always, of course, there are atypical individuals with quirks and foibles of all sorts.

If you have enjoyed your old dog and liked his personality, and still have (sensibly) decided that you don't want a look-alike to replace him, you may find the dog you want within the *group* to which he belonged rather than in the breed itself. For example, if you have lost a Golden Retriever, you would do well to look carefully at the Labradors, black and yellow—both of whom have personalities (I think) among the greatest in dogdom. Or, if you had a fine Fox Terrier but feel that now you could do with a little less enthusiasm, a miniature Schnauzer or a Cairn Terrier might be just what you are looking for. You will fare easier and better, I believe, if you think *group* rather than *breed.*

Inbreeding, overbreeding, and show breeding have produced among the purebreds some hereditary problems that you should be aware of. The Dachshund, for example, is too often prone to posterior paresis. The Pug is very difficult to keep slim. The Scottish Terriers are more likely to have skin troubles than most dogs, and lately there seems to be a cancer problem with them, too. The Pekingese has more eye trouble than most people are prepared to contend with. A short life expectancy is common in all the giant breeds—Great Dane, Saint Bernard, Newfoundland, Great Pyrenees—as is dysplasia. The Boxer is also short-lived. Poodles and Collies have a high incidence of blindness late in life. I used to breed English

Bulldogs, but I gave up because their pushed-in faces caused so many problems.

In fairness, however, I should say that in all of the breeds I have mentioned there are strains that have at least a smaller incidence of the weaknesses I have indicated. Sometimes the problem is serious in only one breeding community. In my area, for instance, personality problems are unfortunately common in the Dalmatians, but where you live they may well be safe and sound. Your old reliable veterinarian, once again, will be your best source of information about the breed you are interested in. He sees hundreds of dogs and he is the first to know when a tendency has become a problem. And while you are talking to him, you might ask him about current prices in the area. He knows what's right and what's outrageous.

Mixed breeds? Mongrels? For me the answer is, why not? If he's a good dog. But you must remember that I am so interested in the dog's personality that I am likely to ignore quirks in his ancestry and even in his appearance. Will Rogers once said that he never met a man he didn't like. That doesn't seem to me to speak well of Rogers's perception, but I admit that I have the same kind of myopic view of dogs. I have rarely seen an ugly dog, and I really don't care much whether he's handsome or not. I just want him to act right.

There is this to be said for mixed breeds: they are relatively free of the genetic problems we have just been talking about. These are generally recessive in mixed breeds and mongrels who are commonly blessed with durable health and what is called—or used to be called—hybrid vigor. Among such dogs it is rare to find a case of retained testicles, certain types of inherited eye problems, umbilical hernias, or dysplasia. We haven't controlled their breeding enough to spoil them.

Size? Big enough to suit you. The right size for you.

And for your circumstances. Not, I hope, a Great Dane in a one-room efficiency apartment or one of the Toys to lope across the great open spaces with you. (There are looming social concerns involved, too, but this is not the platform for that lecture. Sooner or later—and right now is already late—we are going to have to face the problems of population growth, human and animal; environmental pollution; crowding; and the brutal facts of food allocation in a starving world. We should—we must—begin to think now about how many dogs we need, and how many dogs need how many calories.)

Male, female, or altered? As you please. Some like boys, and others like girls. And today more animals than ever before are being neutered. But a great many owners still resist the idea of spaying a bitch and (strangely) they are often even more repelled by the idea of altering a male. Anthropomorphism again, I suppose. But both as your friendly veterinarian and as a person who has had many altered dogs at home, I can assure you that neutering does not change a dog's personality. The operation simply eliminates the sex drive so that the dog neither feels it nor knows that it is missing. You are not, therefore, *depriving* the dog of one of the great pleasures of life. Usually I recommend that the surgery on the male be done about the time he begins to lift his leg to urinate, and on the female when she is about six months old. But you can pick the time. If you want your female to raise one litter, for example, she can be spayed after that. (And here, too, there is a larger social problem which we are not now discussing. Clearly something will have to be done about unwanted pups that have to be destroyed, stray dogs, the population explosion in dogdom.)

Cost? What you can or will or must or should spend. You know that you can get a dog free—a splendid dog. And you also know that you can spend a fortune for a pedigree that reads Ch . . . Ch . . . Ch . . . or for a publicized rarity that will turn heads on Fifth Avenue. Your choice.

There must be a comfortable spot for you somewhere between these extremes.

It is easy to forget and important to remember that there are also maintenance costs. Health care, death, and taxes are all still unavoidable. And food. In these days feeding, which used to be a nothing, can be a substantial expense if you obligate yourself to support a Saint Bernard—and a disaster if you also think that he needs (or deserves) to dine on prime cuts. On the other hand, a candidate for the poorhouse can keep a Chihuahua in luxury. Grooming is a cost that is commonly overlooked. You can brush up your Beagle with the palm of your hand, but unwary and inexperienced buyers of French Poodles are often stunned when they discover what it costs to maintain that chic.

I have seen elaborate studies of the lifetime cost of keeping a dog. If you include all likely or possible expenses from purchase price to cremation costs, if you add in expenses for leashes, toys, haircuts, and kennel wire, if you throw in the cost of keeping him three weeks each year in a boarding kennel while you are off on vacation, if you total up fifteen years of license charges and then add the cost of the food he will consume over that good long life—the lifetime cost of a dog will astound you.

To put it in the vernacular, this figure may seem to you to be either relevant or irrelevant. Lifetime costs of anything—water, newspapers, chewing gum—are shocking. It is undoubtedly more economical to die young—if you can manage it. It's expensive to live. The only question is whether keeping a dog is one of the more pleasurable ways of spending money.

Long-haired or short? Surely you know that a dog sheds twice a year—and sometimes continuously. And surely you know some poor soul who took his Afghan to the country, let him run through the fields and that evening spent hours trying to comb the burrs out of his coat. And finally had to have him clipped to the skin. If you get a dog that showers hair, it may be of some comfort to know that free and easy shedding is considered by some to be a sign of good health in a dog.

And when you have worked through general questions of this sort, you will discover that there are lesser ones—all relating to your own attitudes and preferences, all to be thought out in terms of your own needs and circumstances, all to be decided on the basis of what you think you know about yourself and what you are able to discover about the candidates.

And sometime, with or without this process of introspection, you will decide what kind of dog you want.

Then: Where will you get the dog? Or, to put it another way, where is the best place to get a dog? Or, in the form in which I usually hear the question, is there some way to avoid getting a *bad* dog? Getting the dog may or may not be a problem for you. But next to deciding which is the right dog for you, the step that is most important is getting a good, sound, healthy dog. There is always an imponderable element of luck in buying a pup—a pup in a poke, because nobody can be certain what is hidden under that silky hide. But still, you are not rolling dice. There are things that you can and should do to reduce the risk to a minimum.

If you are thrice lucky, you may have a good friend who wants to give you a good dog. Thrice lucky, I say. First, that he wants to give the dog to you. Second, that it *is* a good dog. And finally, that the good dog is a good dog for *you*. The chances that the offer will satisfy all three conditions are, of course, not good. Everybody has good friends and some of them are generous with pups and sometimes the pups are great. But that the pup should happen to be exactly the kind that you are looking for at that precise moment is the sort of phenomenal luck that seldom materializes. If it should happen to you, take the pup and be forever grateful. Otherwise, refuse. It'll be difficult. When you are looking for a dog, it's hard to turn down a perfectly good free pup just because he isn't ideal. And certainly you don't want to offend a friend. Still, I say, you should refuse. If he is a good friend and if you tell him why you can't accept his offer, the gift giver won't go away mad. The pup will find another home. And you'll find another pup.

Dogs are difficult both to give and to receive. There is an idea that has occasionally been suggested as a solution for people who have lost an old dog and are a little ambivalent about getting a new one. Suppose, the idea goes, suppose that you are getting along toward retirement, that the children have gone off to raise their own families, that you would still like to have a dog but are a little reluctant to assume the responsibility of keeping a dog and going through the whole training routine again. Suppose, instead of doing that, you get a fine pup for your grandchildren. You would see him often when you visited, and the family could bring him to your place and even leave him with you when they were weekending or off on a vacation. You would, in effect, have a *granddog.*

It sounds good—and sometimes, I suppose, it may turn out to be a true inspiration. But if you are tempted to put the idea into practice, I must warn you that it is loaded and dangerous. If you should decide to try it, don't make it a surprise. Talk it over with the parents of the prospective owners. If they agree, have *them* pick the dog. It is nice of you to pay for it, but it is their family and it should be *their* choice, *their* dog. Not yours, even once removed. And when they do get it, don't tell them how to train it any more than you tell them how to bring up their children. It'll be difficult, but you must remember that it is *their* dog.

And don't be certain that the dog will give you all the filial love and respect that a grandfather could want. A widower friend of mine went through all the proper steps and bought exactly the dog that his son and daughter-in-law wanted. They adored the dog and he developed into a perfect animal for them and their two children. The one fault—the *only* fault—that the granddog had was that he wouldn't let "Dad" into the house. He had to be securely locked in the cellar until Grandfather was entrenched in his chair. The dog could then be released, but the old gentleman had to sit tight and the dog watched him like an enemy within the gates throughout the visit. How like a serpent's tooth—but an extreme case, I think.

If you decide to buy a purebred, you'll probably get a pup at a kennel specializing in the breed, preferably one in your own neighborhood. By the time you make up your mind about the kind of dog you want you will know who the local breeders are and, dog talk being as free and irresponsible as it is, you will have learned a good deal about the reputations of the kennel owners and their dogs. The talk will probably do you no harm —if you learn to distinguish between gospel and the gossip which abounds in the breed fanciers' world. In moderation, it may be useful. Some problems, as I have said, are especially prevalent in certain strains, and you should be aware of any such weaknesses that exist in the local breeding lines. And you should have confidence in the breeder. If you have any doubt whatever about how reputable a dealer is, you should look elsewhere for your pup. Even after you have narrowed the field to one or two kennels, there is no harm in asking your veterinarian's opinion. When you are making a long-term investment in affection and companionship, you leave no stone unturned—not even a veterinarian.

Perhaps the healthiest and most responsive pups you can get come from litters that have been raised in the owner's house. They have been part of the family, they have had a lot of handling and affection, they are accustomed to people ways and to the noise and bustle of household activity. In short, they are likely to have had the attention and companionship that kennel dogs often don't get—and they are generally the better for it. Another thing about house pups is that there is a fair chance that you will see the father as well as the mother, and that's a help in judging pups. It's an advantage with purebreds and almost a must with cross-breeds. You will decide on the evidence how well the pups have been cared for and you will want to be assured of the owner's honesty and responsibility. You will also need to be especially careful about such matters as health records and inoculations. But if you find the right pup in the right home, you couldn't do better.

Pet shops pose a problem. It is of no help at all to be told that there are good shops and bad shops. But it is true—and on the whole, I'm afraid, the bad ones are the more numerous. But it is wrong-headed and unfair to assume that there are no reputable pet shops. There are people who would never consider getting a pup at a pet shop. They are convinced that shops are by their nature dishonest, money-grubbing businesses, that the pups are all produced in dog "factories" somewhere, that the shops are dirty, and that the pups are almost sure to be infected with diseases incubated in the store. That's another sweeping generalization, and in this case it is unduly harsh and usually unjustified.

Obviously any shop where such conditions persisted would be out of business in short order. And certainly there are many reputable and long-established businesses that maintain excellent ethical and health standards. There is no cause to condemn all shops because some are dangerously substandard. And there is no immutable reason why you should not get a dog through a pet shop if you know the owner and the reputation of his place—*really* know, not just have a vague impression that he's a nice guy and the surroundings are pleasant. But before you walk into a strange shop to ask how much is the pup in the window—the one with the wag-gel-lee tail—you'd better meditate on the meaning of *caveat emptor.*

Much the same can be said of pounds and shelters, except that they are there to serve a community purpose and not to turn a profit. You can do a good deed by providing a home for one of their animals and you may find a splendid dog that will cost you no more than a small medical fee or a modest contribution. But I must (reluctantly) urge you to be wary of taking a dog from a shelter unless you are certain that it is properly run. In my part of the country, at least, dogs from a large area are gathered into a single facility, and all of them are exposed to the diseases that any of them have. Generally dogs are not inoculated in a pound, and the animals that people get there consequently have a much higher incidence of contagious disease than others. What appears to be a healthy puppy turns out at the end of one incubation period or another to be a very sick little dog—sick even though you may have taken him immediately to your veterinarian and had him inoculated. It is true—happily true—that some shelters are well run and that every puppy is inoculated at least for distemper and hepatitis. And it is true that it is difficult to resist the call of compassion and social conscience. But you will be engaged in a risky kind of charity unless you have firm knowledge that the shelter from which you rescue your dog is properly run.

When you get your pup, you'll want the *pick of the litter,* of course. Everybody does. But what *is* the pick of the litter? By definition, I suppose, it is the best. Or what seems to be the best in a little heap of stumbling, month-old pups, each trying in his own way to solve the problem of moving four out-sized feet in some purposeful sequence. (Not easy. Try it sometime.) In actual practice, the *pick* is a guess, a gamble, the one promissory pup that seems to you to be a tentative step ahead of the others on the way to becoming the dog you want.

But picking a pup is not mere guesswork. At first glance the pups in a litter may seem to be peas in a pod.

They aren't. They are individuals with many differences —genetic, physical, psychological—significant differences which, as I have said, become more evident and more important as the pups grow to maturity. There are clues to be discovered if you are alert and observant enough to see them. Or, to put it more specifically, if you are bright enough to sit down on the floor with the pups long enough to watch the scramble unfold, to see each of the students tackle a problem and tug at it until he wears it out or vice versa.

Physical development is one factor, but only one. You are not likely to pick the smallest of the lot, though I have seen people yield to the urge to rescue a scrawny little fellow who was being trampled by his bedmates. Nor should you snap up the biggest. He might be just an awkward lout with the luck to latch onto a good teat. You'll avoid extremes and choose a good, sound specimen for reasons other than appearance. You will, of course, want a sturdy, well-built pup, but beyond that you will be looking for the slight signs that he is working on the qualities you want in a grown dog.

If you have heard a word that I have said, you will be looking for *personality,* for a candidate with all the cardinal virtues, a small dog who is alert, active, bright, bold, confident, independent, yet gregarious—a paragon. And if you find two such marvels, so much the better. Put the rest away and watch the two together for a little while. Pick them up. Handle them. Inspect them from tip to tail. Then choose from Column A or Column B. Pay the man. Put the dog under your arm and go. And don't look back.

You've got the best dog you could find. You've got the best dog in your house. You've got the best dog you've ever had—since Hector.

Index